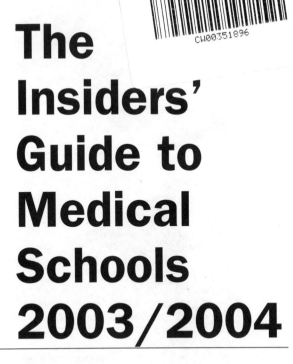

The Insiders' Guide to Medical Schools 2003/2004

The Alternative Prospectus compiled by the BMA Medical Students Committee

Edited by

Alex Almoudaris, Chris Ferguson and Sally Girgis

BMJ
Books

© BMJ Publishing Group 1998, 1999, 2000, 2001, 2002, 2003
BMJ Books is an imprint of the BMJ Publishing Group

First published in 1998
by BMJ Books, BMA House, Tavistock Square,
London WC1H 9JR

First edition 1998
Second edition 1999
Third edition 2000
Fourth edition 2001
Fifth edition 2002
Second impression 2002
Sixth edition 2003

www.bmjbooks.com

British Library Cataloguing in Publication Data

A catalogue record for this book is available from the British Library

ISBN 0 7279 1733 1

Cartoons © Clive Featherstone
Typeset by SIVA Math Setters, Chennai, India
Printed and bound in Spain by Graphycems, Navarra

Contents

Alex Almoudaris is a fifth year intercalating student at Imperial College and was part of the first cohort of the Imperial's new course. He plans to pursue a career in orthopaedics.

Chris Ferguson is a fifth year student at the University of Manchester. He completed an intercalated BSc in infection at the Royal Free Medical School last year. He plans to pursue a career in tropical medicine.

Sally Girgis is Secretary of the Medical Students Committee at the British Medical Association. She is an Australian living in London.

Foreword

Welcome to the sixth edition of *The Insiders' Guide to Medical Schools* – a guide designed to help you make the right decisions when applying to medical school in the UK.

All UK medical schools are included. The authors of each school profile are members and former members of the British Medical Association's Medical Students Committee. Our aim is to provide you with an open and honest insight into the reality of studying medicine at each of our schools. Also included is useful general information and advice about medicine as a career, achieving a place at medical school, and managing your finances as a student.

The last 10 years have been a time of great change for undergraduate medicine. There has been a substantial increase in the number of medical school places available, new medical schools have been formed, and the variety in course structure offered by the different universities has never been greater. With more and more scientific and technological advances being made every day, it is no longer possible to learn "everything" at medical school. Universities are now attempting to equip students with the skills they need to access information and continue to develop professionally long after the graduation ceremony is behind them. Although the core topics to be studied are determined by the General Medical Council, the way in which teaching and learning are approached differs between the individual schools, with some offering a course based mainly on self-directed problem solving and some retaining a more traditional lecture-based curriculum.

Undoubtedly different people are more suited to different styles of learning, and it is important that you use this book, in conjunction with the university prospectuses, to help you choose the kind of institution, course and location that are right for you. Indeed, not everyone is suited to a career in medicine at all, and it is important that you have thought carefully about your own aspirations and dreams before you apply. If you have been influenced predominantly by parental demands or school expectations, then you may suffer an unhappy time both at university and in your future career. Take the opportunities available to visit the medical schools you are most interested in and speak to as many students as you can while you are there in order to canvass their experiences and views. Time spent in careful consideration now will make an instrumental difference to both your enjoyment and your success at medical school.

Despite the heavy workload and increasing cost of studying medicine, medics, as doctors in training, enjoy a very privileged position. We are given the opportunity to work with our patients during some of their most difficult and personal moments, and our course is a unique blend of science and humanities. On completion of the undergraduate course we have the ability to enter into a phenomenally worthwhile and rewarding career in which our primary objective must be to serve. I applaud you on your interest in this great vocation and I wish you the very best for your applications and interviews.

Jennie Ciechan
Chairman
BMA Medical Students Committee

Preface

"The life so short, the craft so long to learn" *Hippocrates on medicine*

Choosing to study medicine is a great undertaking. It will challenge you mentally, physically, emotionally, and financially. If you choose to apply to medical school we feel you should have the most informed choice possible.

This book is a compilation of what we feel you should know, regarding both *what studying medicine really involves* and what characterises the individual medical schools. Each medical school chapter is written by a current medic at that school, hence *The Insiders' Guide*.

This book contains information which, in our experience, students applying to medical school are rarely given, but which with our hindsight is crucial to making *the right choice*. This right choice is not simply the decision as to whether to study medicine or not, but includes thoughts on which medical schools to apply to, what assessment structures will best suit you and the atmosphere in which you will thrive the most. We hope the information in this book will go some way towards helping you make the most suitable choice for you.

Remember: although this is a daunting period, maintain your enthusiasm, remain optimistic and, most importantly of all, pursue your desires to the best of your abilities.

Good luck.

Sally Girgis, Alex Almoudaris and Chris Ferguson

Acknowledgements and contributors

This book is updated every year by the BMA's Medical Students Committee, which represents 13 000 medical students in the UK. Two medical students are elected yearly to the editorial team. If you have any suggestions for ways in which the *Insiders' Guide* could be improved, we'd like to hear them. Email: students@bma.org.uk.

Past editors
Simon Calvert, Deborah Cohen, Lizz Corps, Kristian Mears, Richard Partridge, Kinesh Patel, Jill Spencer, Ian Urmston

Student contributors in the 2003/2004 edition
Alex Almoudaris, Hannah Bayes, Nadia Blunt, Joanna Burgess, Laura Burgess, Laura Buxton, Ben Carrick, Emma Coley, Charlotte Cross, Chris Ferguson, Katie Fletcher, Nick France, Daniel Frith, James Gibson, Jane Graham, Ian Harwood, Peter Hersey, Neema Jaberi, Bhanu Janagan, Elizabeth Kingston, Nickolas Papadakos, Victoria Parker, Amit Parmar, Declan Quinn, Will Redmond, Balvinder Sagoo, Stephan Sanders, Robin Sanderson, Faheem Shakur, Gabriel Shaya, Alice Sisson, Fiona Stonely, Nicholas Thomas and Christopher Windle

Cartoons created by
Clive Featherstone

Editorial assistance
Eleanor Babbington, Felicity Espley, Neil Gadhok, Sally Girgis, Kim Lenart, Shalini Patel

With apologies to any contributors we may have accidentally missed out.

Meet Mikey

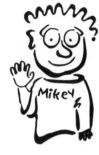

Hi, I'm Mikey.

I'm here to give you the inside information on life as a medical student and a career in medicine This book is split into two parts:

Part 1 contains insiders' information designed to help you decide whether medicine is the right choice for you, how to choose the right medical school, how to apply, and other important issues you should know.

Part 2 gives valuable information and views about every medical school in the UK. The strength of this book lies in the fact that it has been written by students, for students. It provides opinions that are not always found in medical school prospectuses or in the UCAS handbook. Each medical school entry has been divided for ease into three categories: Academia, Sport and Social Life. Students have also provided insight into the "great" and "bad" things about each school. To make flicking through easier, the following symbols will appear throughout the book:

 Education

 Welfare

 Sports and social

 Great things about the medical school

 Bad things about the medical school

Now, it won't surprise you that student life differs radically from one university to the next. What may surprise you is that each medical school offers a course which is to some extent unique. Medics, more than anyone else, can give you the lowdown on the distinguishing features you may want to consider. A book like this could never claim to be totally objective or definitive about all the differences and similarities, or strengths and weaknesses between the medical schools. Every effort has been made to ensure that the opinions of the medical students who contributed to the book are based on factual information. Take the opinions offered here into account and we strongly recommend you use this information alongside other materials you will have collected (for example, prospectuses or the opinions of others) as you draw up your shortlist of where to apply.

REMEMBER:

☑ Read the medical school/university prospectus
☑ Read the alternative prospectus
☑ Visit the medical school (some have open days)
   and the town or city
☑ Visit the medical school website

GOOD LUCK!

Part 1
Insiders' information

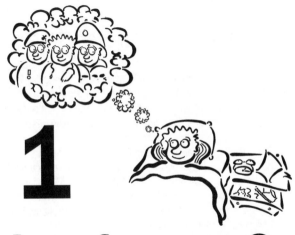

1

Is medicine for you?

Ask the average student why they are applying to study medicine and they'll probably tell you it's because they enjoy science and want to help people. Probe a little deeper and they may mention ideas such as money, and the fact that they are expected to get good A-level grades. Medicine may even command a certain amount of kudos and possibly sex appeal!

Although trends may be changing, doctors have traditionally been held in high regard by the general public, which many students find an appealing prospect. A 2002 MORI public opinion poll reported that doctors were the most trusted profession. However, with this respect come responsibility and pressure: one only has to read a small selection of newspapers to see that doctors are a major focus of media attention and public interest. Not all of the resulting coverage is favourable or fair.

Knowing that you are under constant scrutiny, and not always from people who understand clinical medicine, adds to the stresses of the job. As a doctor you will be faced with difficult decisions involving ethical and clinical dilemmas, and these situations can be very stressful. There are also many unpleasant tasks, like breaking bad news or dealing with abusive patients or relatives. Curing patients is fulfilling and exciting – it happens regularly in some specialties – but there will be many patients you can't cure, many symptoms that can't be controlled, and many "worried well" who can't be persuaded that they are not in fact ill.

The number of people applying to study medicine in 2003 has risen by 28·1% in the last 12 months to 14 040 (this has been partly due to the expansion of the number of medical schools in the last few years). Despite the increasing number of places there is still a shortage of doctors in the UK, which means there are more than enough jobs to go round.

Salaries for junior doctors have increased significantly over the last few years and are set to continue rising. Junior doctors can be paid an annual salary of up to £34,000 (before tax), but the workload can be very demanding. The wage varies to reflect the working pattern, the intensity of work and the antisocial nature of the post. As you become more senior in your chosen field, pay improves, often with the scope for private income. However, if your only aim in medicine is to make endless amounts of money, to prance around in a white coat looking like a star from a TV drama, or to prove how able you are to pass exams, forget it. There are many easier ways to make money and the work is only occasionally glamorous. Application and dedication to patient care and learning are far more important attributes than the ability to continually pass difficult exams.

The British Medical Association (BMA) is the doctors' trade union and professional organisation. It has sought, in negotiation with government, to reduce the hours of work and improve doctors' terms and conditions of service. The BMA's Junior Doctor Committee has agreed the new pay deal for junior doctors. The deal has removed overtime rates of pay, which were at one time less than the normal hourly rate. The BMA is continuing negotiations to bring working conditions in line with the European Working Time Directive.

To follow particular career directions in medicine you will need to study and sit postgraduate exams (after qualifying). It is vital that you continue your medical education if you are to keep your skills and knowledge up to date. It's a long haul, and requires a commitment and devotion that far exceed any financial rewards. Whatever combination of reasons has made you choose medicine, remember it is a vocation. Those who enter medical school with a strong commitment to work hard, learn, and serve patients to their best ability are the people most likely to find life as a doctor richly rewarding and stimulating.

The medical profession is increasingly diverse, with ethnic minorities comprising 30% of the intake to medical school. It would be untrue to say that racial and sexual discrimination does not occur in medical schools or the health service, but the BMA, NHS Executive and all medical schools are active in promoting equal opportunities.

Many gay, lesbian and bisexual applicants are unsure whether their sexuality may affect their future career. Although some within the profession may hold unsympathetic views, they are a decreasing minority. Be reassured that gay, lesbian and bisexual doctors are found at all grades, across all specialties. Although many are happy to be open with colleagues about their sexuality, others still prefer to keep their personal lives private.

The Human Rights Act, which came into effect in 2001, offers greater protection to people who are not treated equally. The GMC also states that doctors should not show prejudice. The law and the intentions of professional bodies are laudable, but tackling the issue of diversity with respect to age, disability, ethnic origin, gender and sexual orientation is challenging. Details of support for people who feel that they are being treated unfairly can be found in the Further Information appendix of this book.

Don't be surprised if you have any doubts about studying medicine. Many potential medics will also be flirting with the idea of pharmacy, law, veterinary science and other courses. Speak to some doctors – your own GP might be a start – or arrange some work experience at your local hospital. Entering medicine is not a decision to be taken lightly or for the wrong reasons.

Finally, the choice to study medicine should be your own. It will be you who finds the force of character to spend endless nights before exams revising. It will be you who needs to find the capacity to carry on studying for up to three years after the rest of your school friends have graduated and begun earning. Ultimately, the choices you make now will determine the rest of your working life. If you feel others are making these choices for you, now is the time to muster the courage to face up to those who put these pressures on you.

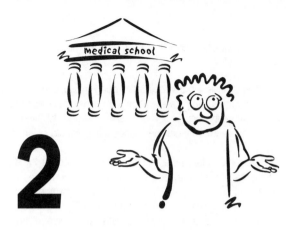

2

Life as a medical student

How am I going to be taught?

In the past, there was a view that medical students spent their first couple of years cramming a vast amount of knowledge without ever seeing a patient, and then emerged brainwashed, unable to think and unable to communicate.

If this ever was the case, it is now certainly a thing of the past. Recommendations in the General Medical Council (GMC) report called *Tomorrow's Doctors* encouraged medical schools to reduce the emphasis on learning factual information and concentrate much more on developing the skills and attitudes needed to become a doctor. The report also recommended the introduction of special study modules (SSMs) to give students the chance to undertake projects of their own choosing. Alongside this, the GMC encouraged schools to adopt a more "problem-based" learning approach to teaching, where facts are taught within a framework of real-life clinical scenarios.

Developing research skills and encouraging intellectual curiosity and enthusiasm for learning are now as important as knowledge. The majority of medical schools have already changed their curricula so that older courses (in which science and clinical practice were taught separately) have given way to more "integrated" curricula. In other words, instead of learning subjects separately – for example anatomy, biochemistry, and physiology ("subject-based teaching") – students are more likely to learn about respiration, reproduction, diet, and metabolism in a more "systems-based" approach.

In most schools, students will have some regular contact with clinicians and patients from the outset. The early years still have less clinical content and more lecture and laboratory teaching, but the traditional preclinical/clinical divide is dying. An important effect of these changes is that students need to be much more responsible for their own studies, and lots of self-motivation is needed. New

5

clinical skills laboratories have been introduced in many schools so that students can practise procedures and take exams on dummies. This helps to build confidence before going on the wards and meeting patients. The balance between lectures, problem-based learning, SSMs and clinical exposure will vary between schools and should be spelt out in each prospectus.

Clinical work takes place in local teaching hospitals and district general hospitals (DGHs), which can be many miles away from the medical school. These "attachments" take you out of town, but getting away from the big city hospitals can give you the chance to be more useful and learn more. Most schools provide free accommodation within the hospitals if commuting is not practicable. Some schools will even allow overseas attachments in addition to the elective (covered in more detail below).

You can interrupt most courses by studying for an extra "intercalated" degree. This is normally a medical science degree (BSc, BMedSci) undertaken during an extra year (or two) of study. It is commonly taken after the second or third year, and entry policies vary between schools. It is compulsory in some, actively encouraged in others, and some allow it by invitation only. In some schools where it is voluntary, as many as 50% of each year group intercalate at some stage in their studies. The main consideration to extending an already long course to complete an intercalated degree is the issue of financing the extra 12 months. At some schools and in some situations tuition fees for the intercalated degree year are paid for, but you will still need to finance maintenance for an extra year. Further details about intercalated degrees can be found in Chapter 3.

During the final years of the course there is normally a medical elective. This is a period of weeks or months when students travel to a specialist clinic or hospital attachment of their own choice. This can be in the UK, but many use the opportunity to go overseas and learn about medicine in the developing world, a particular disease or condition, or another system of healthcare delivery. Electives can be the high point of medical student life. Students who get themselves organised early enough can usually find enough funding for an elective to help avoid paying for all of it themselves. Many combine the elective with some extra travel and a holiday. The length of time available for the elective(s) depends on the medical school. Normally information is held locally about where students have been in recent years, which might help you decide where to go. Missionary, voluntary and charity organisations can sometimes help you find a suitable clinic or hospital to visit, or academic departments at your medical school may have some prepackaged electives with fellow institutes abroad.

But I'm squeamish!

As you would imagine, there is a fair amount of blood and gore in medicine at various stages (for example physiology practicals, postmortems, dissection, and taking blood). Many students become used to this remarkably quickly. For others, it may take longer. It may surprise you to know that some doctors are still squeamish after many years of practice. If you are very concerned about how you might react, try to arrange some appropriate work experience at your local hospital.

I've heard it's really hard work!

The GMC puts great emphasis on skills and attitudes rather than the traditional rote learning of huge amounts of facts. Increasingly, formal lectures are out and problem-based integrated learning is in!

However, there are still exams. Many medical schools examine by continuous assessment and have rearranged the finals so that they are taken over a longer period rather than all at once. This has been a sensible development and has reduced a lot of the periodic pressure. Some, however, would argue that this has only spread the pressure throughout the year; the increased number of exams can lead to exam fatigue and at some schools with more traditional courses, "finals" are still dreaded.

Friends studying for other degrees may have as many hours timetabled per week as you'll have in one day – and you'll have to study in the evenings. In fact, attendance at lectures/practicals/clinical sessions can last from 9 am until 5 pm every day, and a register might be taken. Medics have to compare this with other students, who might only have four hours of lectures a week! Additional time is needed for personal study and revision. Exams also demand time and energy for preparation.

Also, graduates from other, shorter courses may be in a job and earning more money than you will be when you qualify, and you may still have two more years of unpaid study left before you get a salary!

Being a medical student is enjoyable but hard work. It involves many hours in lectures, tutorials, practicals, clinics and wards. It soon becomes apparent that the commitments and expectations are far greater than applicants might have expected, and also far greater than those of your friends on other degree courses. Depending on the medical school you choose, different portions of your study time will be allocated to different teaching methods or subjects. More information about varying elements of the course can be found in Chapter 3.

Is it fun?

Despite all these pressures, medical students have no trouble being sporty and sociable. In fact, we often excel at both. There is a wide mixture of students at every medical school and every group will contain a range of public school and state school, working class and middle class, medical family and non-medical family type backgrounds You will be able to pursue your non-course interests as well as your studies. "Work hard and play hard" is the maxim that unites medical students and the medical profession has an enviable community spirit – a "we're all in it together" attitude. Year groups are generally large (200+) and, because everyone is doing the same course, you get to know your colleagues very quickly and very well. The downside of this is that medical students sometimes have a reputation for not mixing with students on other courses. It is also why we have the enviable reputation for the best social life! The common shared purpose amongst those studying medicine makes for a closeness, which is one of the best aspects of life as a medical student.

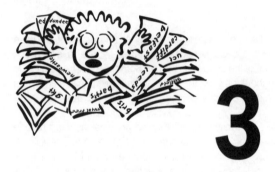

3

Choosing the right medical school

Information for all applicants

Numerous factors influence which medical schools you may decide to apply for. In this chapter we have summarised a number of important areas we think you should take into consideration before making a decision.

Education

Although all students need to reach the same standard by the time they graduate, courses at different medical schools can vary considerably in the way that this is achieved. More often than not the courses on offer are subject to change, and many of us at medical school are on different courses from those outlined in the original prospectus. Don't, whatever you do, get bogged down in the details of individual courses. You'll just get confused. However, it may be worthwhile considering the following areas.

Teaching

There are two broad teaching methods, which may be used on their own in some schools whereas others offer a mix of the two. "Traditional" teaching relies heavily on lectures and practicals, with a large portion of the week devoted to didactic teaching where students are in lecture theatres for long periods.

Problem-based learning (PBL) is the more recent approach, and usually has fewer timetabled commitments. Commonly, students work in small groups and discuss patient case studies, from which they form study agendas for the coming week. Students then work through their own study objectives, which are supplemented with laboratory sessions such as pathology and anatomy in the preclinical years, and maybe attendance at outpatient clinics in the clinical years. With the PBL approach, it is essential that students sustain a significant amount of self-motivation.

Anatomy teaching has also seen many changes in recent years, with the dissection of cadavers by students being replaced, partly or fully, with demonstration sections (or prosections) dissected by staff prior to class. This is often less gruesome and doesn't necessitate students "getting their hands wet".

Assessment

The type of assessment varies significantly between schools. Commonly used methods include multiple choice question papers, essay papers, short answer questions, computer examinations, literature review papers and case studies ... and many more. Some schools even have final exams in the penultimate year. Other schools have a greater amount of continuous assessment, which reduces the impact of finals at the end of the course.

When choosing which medical schools to apply for, decide whether you would prefer exams and assessments spread out, or whether you would prefer to wait until everything fits into place at the last moment before sitting exams.

Intercalated degrees

This is where medical students can obtain a Bachelor of Science degree for undertaking an extra year of study, once they have completed at least two years of their medical training. These degrees can be undertaken in a variety of subjects related to medicine and provide an opportunity for students to pursue further study in an area they are interested in. UK medical schools take a variety of approaches to intercalated degrees. In some (although this is a disappearing approach) the extra degree is open only to the academic high-flyers, some offer courses to almost any medical student, and at others it is compulsory. If you anticipate being interested in some extra in-depth research leading to a qualification or if you think you might like to follow an academic or teaching career, then think about this before you apply. Many medical schools also allow students to study for the extra degree within other faculties of the university or at other universities.

Special study modules (SSM) and electives

Different schools devote various portions of the course to studying areas of special interest to individual students, and also to overseas work placements. Some medical schools will allow two- to four-week SSMs in subjects such as history of medicine, medicine and art, and modern languages. There is even a move to allow students to take SSMs in subjects unrelated to medicine! Schools also offer students an opportunity to spend a longer part of the course (around two months) anywhere in the world to experience medicine in a foreign healthcare setting. The exact nature of these placements varies between schools, and may be worth looking into.

Welfare

Student support

Pastoral support systems should be in place at all universities. Some universities will provide support through the medical faculty as well as from the main campus. Many schools have in-house counselling services too. In the first few weeks at many universities freshers are allocated "mummies and daddies" to help them settle in, and most schools allocate students to personal tutors, should problems arise.

Accommodation

The accommodation the university provides and where it is located will have an important effect on your experience of university: remember you will spend a large portion of your time there. Important questions to ask include

- Is accommodation provided for the first year?
- Are meals provided or is the residence self-catering?
- Is the accommodation on campus, and if not, how far away is it?
- How expensive is the accommodation for the first and subsequent years?

Placements

Most schools will send you away from the main university base for some modules. The distances involved can vary significantly. Are you the type who enjoys travelling and seeing different parts of the country or would you rather stay nearer your new home town and spend less on travel?

Sports and social 🏆

All medical schools offer medics' sports teams. Only students studying medicine will be able to represent these clubs. As almost all medical schools are now part of larger universities you will also be able to play for the university side. However, you tend to find that most medics pride themselves on playing for the medics. The camaraderie and social life are unrivalled and a constant envy of non-medics.

As some universities organise social weekends before the start of freshers' term this is a great way of making friends even before other freshers arrive. The comfort of walking into the bar on the first evening of term and recognising a friendly face from such a weekend relieves some of the initial anxiety of leaving home and making new friends.

The only limit on the number of teams you can join is the amount of time you are willing to devote. Most students wonder how medics can study during the day, train in the evenings and play matches week in and week out: the answer is that you develop good time management skills.

One beauty of medics' sports is that all skill levels are catered for, and as you progress in your medical career you may find you take on more responsibility for your club, from organising the mundane – kit – to the extravagant – tours to South America for the water polo team, for example!

Do get involved, try something new, excel at something old, but most importantly, ENJOY IT!

4

Choosing the right medical school

For graduate and premedical/foundation course applicants

Not everyone knows from an early age that medicine is the career for them. Many students gain A-levels or even degrees before deciding to pursue a career in medicine. This section gives course information for these students, along with details of application procedures.

Graduate entry programmes (GEP)

Nowadays more and more entrants to medical school have already completed an undergraduate degree and may be eligible to undertake a four-year fast-track graduate entry programme (GEP). In fact, many of the government's planned new places are being reserved for graduates as schools develop graduate-only courses. Medical schools view graduates as reliable and likely to "stay the course". These mature students have done something else with their lives – often another degree – before taking the plunge into medicine and, it can be argued, have spent more time assessing whether they really want to be a doctor. In some schools as many as 15% of students are graduate entrants, and the staff are used to dealing with their different needs.

By September 2003, nine medical schools will offer graduate entry programmes. These courses vary in their entry requirements: Leicester/Warwick and Oxford require a good honours degree (first or upper second class) in science or a health-related subject, whereas the other five schools will accept a good honours degree in any subject. In addition, some schools require applicants to undertake an entrance exam, the results of which are used to offer interviews. Some more details on the various graduate entry programmes can be seen in the table below, but students are encouraged to contact the relevant universities for more information.

University	Places	Course details
Birmingham	40	Four-year medical course open to graduates of life science subjects. Students are taught in a separate stream for the first two years, before joining the specialty clinical rotations of the fourth and fifth years of the current five-year MBChB degree
Bristol	19	Four-year medical course requiring a 2.1 BSc in biomedical science
Cambridge	20	Four-year medical course open to graduates of **any** discipline. All candidates are required to take the Medical and Veterinary Admissions Test (MVAT)
Leicester/ Warwick	164	Four-year medical course open to graduates of biological sciences commenced 1999 at the Warwick site
	64	Four-year medical course open to graduates of health sciences commenced 2002 at the Leicester site
Liverpool	40	Four-year medical course open to graduates of approved biomedical disciplines or health or social care professions due to commence in 2003
Newcastle	95	Four-year medical course open to graduates of **any** discipline. No entrance examination necessary
Nottingham	90	Four-year medical course open to graduates of **any** discipline due to commence 2003. Applicants have to complete the GAMSAT test, which is designed to ensure that entrants have the requisite knowledge and reasoning skills
Oxford	30	Four-year graduate entry course for biological science graduates. After a special two-year transition course taught at the hospital site, with the support of college-based tutorials, the accelerated programme leads into the final two years of the standard clinical course. Applicants have to complete a written test
St Bart's	40	Four-year medical course open to graduates with a science or health-related studies degree due to commence 2003. The admissions process for the GEP is currently under consideration but is likely to include a structured interview
St George's	70	Four-year medical course open to graduates in **any** discipline. Applicants have to complete the GAMSAT test (this tests knowledge, reasoning skills and communication across a range of disciplines). Those who perform well in the test are offered an interview

Most self-funding students and many graduate entrants will incur higher levels of debt than their younger colleagues. However, finances should not put you off applying to medical school if you have a true desire to become a doctor. Although many schools do not normally consider applicants over 30 years of age, some graduate programmes have no upper age limit! Don't forget that competition for graduate places may be tough: at St George's in 2002, 500 students sat the GAMSAT; of these only 120 were invited for interview, and only 60 were offered a place on the course.

Premedical courses

Most medical degree courses last five years, but some are six and include a compulsory BSc year. In addition to these five or six years, some schools offer an additional foundation year, also known as the premedical year. This year, which is intended as a foundation year in basic sciences, gives students with good non-science A-level grades (and some non-science graduates, if there is not an appropriate graduate entry programme) a way into the medicine degree course.

There are significant variations in the way these courses are taught and organised, and the exact nature of the premedical course varies from school to school. At some schools, students who complete the year successfully can apply to join the medical degree course, whereas at others there is automatic transfer to the first year of the five-year course.

Premedical courses may be taught within the medical faculty or in other university departments. Exemptions from parts of the course may be offered if that subject has already been studied to a sufficient level, and some schools offer a choice of subject studied. In addition, certain schools also specify that particular science subjects are needed at GCSE/Standard Grade level.

Medical schools offering premedical courses are listed opposite, along with some course details.

University	Places	Course details
Belfast	5	Course for students with more broadly based qualifications than A-levels, e.g. Scottish Highers or Irish Leaving Certificate. Students attend first-year courses in chemistry, physics and biological science
Bristol	10	The premed year is spent studying the equivalent of A-levels in chemistry, biology and physics. Premedical students study alongside predental students
Cardiff	16	The premedical is a modular course. A core programme centres on the sciences, but modules are selected according to each student's prior qualifications. There are also optional components chosen by the student in areas such as humanities, health sciences, psychology or languages. Assessment consists of a combination of coursework, class tests and end of module examinations
Dundee	Usually no more than 10	Dundee's premed students join with first-year BSc courses in chemistry, biology and physics
Edinburgh	No set number	The premed year consists of following courses from the first-year biological sciences course. The particular choice of courses depends on the individual student's qualifications
GKT	35	Designed for students who do not meet subject requirements for the full medical programme, for example those with arts A-levels. The course covers biology, chemistry, physics, and maths. Students study alongside those taking BSc degrees
Manchester	20	Students learn fundamentals of biology, physics, and chemistry in an environment which has a relevance to clinical medicine. This is achieved with problem-based learning cases, theatre events, and skills sessions. Assessment is at the end of each of the two semesters and includes multiple choice paper, slide-based multiple choice, computing exam, laboratory-based skills test, a seen patient case, and an unseen patient case
Newcastle	10–15	Students study a combination of chemistry, biological sciences, and medical data handling. GCSE passes in maths, English, and at least one other science subject are needed. Scottish students need to have Standard Grade chemistry
Sheffield	15	The bespoke course is at Barnsley College and has been revamped in the last two years. There are visits to the medical physics, clinical chemistry and anaesthetic departments of a local hospital. Additionally, students gain basic scientific knowledge through studying biology, chemistry and physics. MBChB foundation students are full members of the University of Sheffield. Assessment is at end of semester; written examinations occur in each subject area, making up the bulk of the marks. The remainder of the assessment is in-course practical work

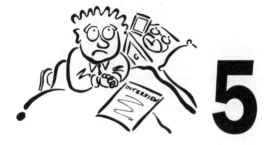

5

Applying to medical school

Important information to increase your chances of getting an interview, and receiving an offer

Entrance requirements

Most medical schools require students to get A or B grades (mainly As) in at least three full A-level subjects (discounting general studies) or five Scottish Highers. Many schools also require the Scottish Certificate of Sixth Year Studies from applicants educated in Scotland. The entry requirements have gone up, and have remained high despite the drop in applicants. The average requirement is now AAB (AAABB). Chemistry is usually a compulsory requirement because the principles of chemistry are the key to understanding medical biochemistry, and it would be difficult to teach to the required standard during the course. Surprisingly, many schools don't insist on biology, although many medics have it as one of their A-levels. In most schools medical teaching covers elementary biology, and there may be supplementary classes for non-biologists during the first year.

Traditionally, the other subjects studied at A-level are sciences or mathematics, but many medical schools now acknowledge that students who pursue other subjects at school are not disadvantaged when they begin studying medicine. Some schools accept applications from students taking chemistry, another science subject and an arts A-level. It is essential to check with each school before you make your final choices: don't rely upon what others have chosen before if your choices are a non-typical combination. Where possible, the key facts box for each medical school reflects that school's requirements of the AS-levels.

Health status

In addition to academic qualifications, you will also have to fulfil certain health-related entry requirements. Individual schools have different requirements, about which they will inform you if your application is successful, but in general you will need **immunity against rubella and TB** if you don't already have it. You will also need to **prove your hepatitis B status** before admission. Hepatitis B carriers are excluded from performing blood exposure-prone procedures, and in the unlikely event that a medical school applicant tests e antigen positive they will almost certainly be refused admission to the course. Contact your GP as soon as possible to arrange for these tests to be done!

The UCAS form ... the first step

Medical schools only accept applications made through the Universities and Colleges Admissions Service (UCAS). Read through the *UCAS Handbook* and follow the advice closely. Make several drafts of your UCAS form before finalising your application. Your careers tutor at school or college will be able to help you fill in the form, but remember to make it accurate and legible.

The most important part of the form is the personal statement. This is your chance to stand out from the crowd and make the admissions tutors want to interview you. What you write will go a long way towards determining how many medical schools offer you an interview or a place. The comments below apply equally to electronic and paper applications.

You can expect – not surprisingly – that the medical school will want to know why you want to study medicine and, as there is so much competition, you must seize this opportunity to demonstrate your commitment to joining the profession. For example, you may want to try to describe what drives you to pursue a career in medicine, and how you have gone about trying to understand what this career will entail. However, don't take too much space to do this, as it will be at the expense of other important information. The challenge is to do this effectively with supporting evidence of a well-balanced character, for example, the hospital portering job, regularly visiting a local old people's home, captaining the school netball team, or editing the school magazine. These examples will prove to them that you are a good candidate and that you are well rounded in your interests.

It should be clear from the information supplied by your school or college whether you have the potential to get the grades, so the personal statement must show you as a potential asset to the medical school and, later, the medical profession. They will be looking for

- Signs of good interpersonal skills
- Evidence of a social life
- Details of your interests/hobbies
- Any notable achievements.

You could mention

- Sports achievements
- Academic prizes

- Organisational or supervisory positions of responsibility
- Voluntary work, part-time work
- Musical or travel interests
- Projects you have particularly enjoyed or unusual hobbies.

If you are deferring entry for a year you should explain how you are going to use your time.

There is no need to explain your choice of A-levels unless you have something interesting to say about them, for example: "I am studying computing as an A-level as I think it may lie at the heart of medicine in the future". Don't be afraid of making bold comments as long as you can justify them. They also offer signposts for interviewers that can be prepared for before an interview (see interview section below).

If you are called for an interview the panel will question you on the contents of this section, so don't lie or exaggerate your interests or achievements. Remember, you may be asked to talk about any of the things you mention, so be truthful – it will probably show very quickly if you have embellished too much!

Admissions staff read through hundreds of UCAS forms, and if yours stands out then you will have a better chance of being called for interview. The admissions tutor will want to know that you are prepared for what a career in medicine entails, and that you have realistic expectations, so by the time you post your application form you should have done your research and thinking.

You can use this book to help you decide which schools to apply to, but don't put an overt preference in the application. Another medical school may dismiss your application if they think that you will turn down their offer, and if you change your mind you will have limited your options. Also, think carefully about how your statement will appear to an admissions tutor reading it in his or her office. If you express a passionate interest in Premiership football an admissions tutor at Peninsula might think you would not enjoy being miles from any of the top clubs and not offer you an interview. Equally, an application to a Scottish medical school might appear eminently sensible from a student interested in Ceilidh dancing.

When to apply

Apply as early as possible, but don't rush your application form and remember to submit it well before the appropriate deadlines. The UCAS guide and website give you all the details. You can submit your application electronically. You may receive replies from medical schools virtually as soon as you apply or you may be kept waiting until the last week that offers can be made. Some schools may make a conditional offer on your application alone, whereas others will conduct many rounds of interviews before they make offers or rejections. You may think you have been forgotten – this is very unlikely, but it does happen. If you are in doubt, and the deadline is approaching, contact the admissions office. You can arrange for UCAS to acknowledge receipt of your form, and you will be given an application number so you can check progress if you feel it is taking too long. Admissions offices will be very busy during this time, but a telephone call may put your mind at ease even if they can't give you a decision on your application.

Open days and further information

It is very important that you find out as much as possible about the medical schools that you are considering applying to. In Part 2 of this book we give you admission information and views and opinions for you to consider. Only by visiting the school and reading the prospectus and any alternative guides will you be able to assess the atmosphere and whether you will enjoy studying there. Remember, no one knows what life at medical school is like better than those already there. Don't be afraid to approach us: we are generally a friendly bunch and would be more than happy to chat over a coffee about any aspect of medical school life.

Open days will help you decide whether you would prefer a medical school that is part of a larger university, on a campus or spread across a town, in a big city or near the countryside, and where you'd like to live should you accept a place there. It will also allow you to talk to the medics who are already there. Starting university can be a daunting experience, but if you know what to expect then you will be much more at ease. If you can't afford the travel expenses, get a group together and ask if your school or college will sponsor a minibus or take a coach to an open day. Most open days take place in the summer after the students have had their exams. It is better to go early before the students go on vacation, although there are clinical students milling around all year. Well-organised open days have a welcoming team to escort visitors from the station, and organise events, talks, tours, displays, and demonstrations. However, organisation varies greatly from school to school. Some medical schools run intensive open days during which you may have sample lectures.

There are courses run commercially, giving application advice and an insight into life as a medical student. These can be expensive but may be a good way of helping you decide whether medicine is the right choice for you. Your careers tutor might be able to help you find out about these courses and open days.

If you cannot attend an open day there are a number of people you could write to. The Students Union can deal with enquiries and may have promotional material that it could send you. The Medical Faculty office should also be able to supply you with the name of the president of the Medical Society, the student group responsible for representing medics and organising sports and social events, so you can contact the students directly. BMA student representatives are always happy to answer questions, and they may be contacted through the medical school or via the BMA Medical Students Committee (see Further information).

The interview

If you are called to an interview, make sure you have done your homework.

Interviewers will be looking at your UCAS form for inspiration. They will probably be interested in what is special and unusual (but not weird) about you: they would be fascinated to find out what drove you to do a llama herding course in South America during your gap year – tell them! Reread your personal statement and anticipate the kinds of questions you might be asked. This is where your personal statement and your interview should mesh. Place signposts in your personal statement that interviewers can pick up on and question you about. Remember, they may be interviewing 40 people in one day, and you can make it easier for them by doing this. You should also keep up to date with medical news stories and developments, as these may be the subject of some questioning.

Dress smartly and arrive in good time. If you are going to be shown around the medical school, remember that this is an opportunity to ask current students any questions you might have. Don't feel obliged to ask any questions in the interview, and don't ask questions which are already answered in the prospectus. In some ways an interview is a chance for the medical school to assess the potential it has recognised in your application form. It is not an academic test. Treat it as an opportunity to show that you are serious about your career choice, and that you will be a future asset to the profession.

Most importantly, enjoy your interview. It is an opportunity for the panel to get a feel for the sort of person you are. If you don't agree with something then say so, as long as you can justify your disagreement logically and concisely.

What if I don't get in?

The number of applicants to study medicine dropped more than 3% in 2000 to 9291, but increased in 2001 to 10 958. In spite of this and the increased number of places, medical schools in the UK are still vastly oversubscribed. There are often 10 applicants for each place, and only a small fraction of them will make it to interview, selected on the basis of their UCAS forms and references; even fewer will get a place. Oxford and Cambridge have fewer applicants per place, which might mean that, although the academic requirements are high, you stand a slightly greater chance of at least being called to interview. However, not getting a place to read medicine is simply a reflection of the pressure on places and not a great indictment of your character and abilities. Even if you maximise your chances of being selected for interview, you may still be unsuccessful in your application.

You need to know what to do next. First, think long and hard! Do you still want to study medicine? Medical schools try to select people who will make good doctors and who have the right ability and motivations for studying medicine, but even so some students choose to leave mid-course and others fail exams. The interview panel has a responsibility to make the right decision for the medical school, and you have a responsibility to yourself and your potential future patients to make sure you are making the correct choice. Examine your reasons for wanting to study medicine. If in doubt, or if you have felt pushed in the direction of medicine, it might be better to look at different courses or careers.

If you still want to study medicine, then start by asking yourself why you weren't successful in your application. Did you get an interview? If you did, your school might be able to get some feedback from the medical school. This is unlikely to be in depth, but might give you some useful information. Discuss the prospect of your chances with teachers. Reflecting on your disappointment at this stage may prove difficult, but it is in your interests to be honest and realistic. Think about the possibility of following another course, whether in a related field – for example physiology, pharmacy, physiotherapy, biochemistry – or something totally unrelated. Most universities offer places on degree courses through "clearing". If your grades are good then many other courses will be open to you. It is possible to reapply to read medicine, but some schools will only consider a second application if you applied there first time round. If you do reapply, your A-level results should be at least as good as the estimates that your school originally made. There are some schools that will consider candidates who are resitting. Save your own time and energies by asking your preferred schools if they would accept an application from you. This could prevent you from wasting future UCAS choices. It is only advisable to resit exams if you are sure about getting A grades the second time around or if there were extenuating circumstances, such as bereavement or serious illness, in the months preceding your A-levels first time around.

There are a growing number of places available for graduates to read medicine, which means that you could do a degree and see after graduation whether you still want to become a doctor. Graduates usually follow the full undergraduate medical course unless they can be exempted from part of it because of the nature of their first degree (for example, biochemistry or dentistry). Graduates with a purely arts background at A-level or degree could try to take a medical foundation year (premed year) before the medical course proper. This is not available at all institutions. Many schools don't normally consider applicants over 30 years of age. Graduate entry, however, is one of the ways into a career as a doctor. The BMA, and many other interested parties, have recognised the desirability of graduate entry and, as more places are being reserved for graduates, it is sensible to consider this route as an option.

Gap years

Many sixth-form students defer entry to university for 12 months. Gap years are looked on favourably by most colleges and universities. Most, however, expect you to use the time profitably by working and/or travelling. It is important that you check the medical school's attitude before you apply if you intend to defer entry. Time out between school and university is not just for those who have the money for a "round the world" air ticket: a well-planned gap year will give you time to think about how to get through university and let you assess what you want to get out of the next five or more years. Time spent well will boost your confidence and broaden your experience. This can have a very positive effect on your performance. Student debt is increasing all the time. You could try to save some money and be in better financial shape for your eventual university career. A gap year may also be used to gain some more work experience in healthcare, although there is no need to overdo it, assuming that you gained some experience prior to applying to medical school.

Note: A minority of colleges at Oxford and Cambridge don't approve of gap years. It is best to check the attitude of the individual college(s) you are thinking of applying to.

Mature students

More and more applicants to medical school nowadays are mature students. Medical schools often view mature students as reliable and likely to "stay the course". These applicants have often achieved another degree or worked in professions allied to medicine, such as nursing, and many argue that these students have spent more time assessing whether they really want to be a doctor before taking the plunge into medicine. In some schools as many as 15% of students are mature students, and the staff are used to dealing with their different needs; in other schools older students are a rarity. Depending on their academic background, mature students may be eligible to join one of the fast-track graduate courses, whereas others may have to complete a foundation or premedical year. In these cases it is essential students contact the admissions department of the medical schools to find out if there are specific entrance requirements. Graduate entry programmes (GEP) and premedical courses are discussed in more detail in Chapter 4.

A large proportion of mature students will be self-funding if they have previously completed undergraduate degrees, and consequently are likely to incur higher levels of debt than their younger colleagues. However, finances should not put you off applying to medical school if you are motivated and have a true desire to study medicine and become a doctor.

Students with disabilities

The Disability Discrimination Act 1995 requires universities and medical schools to take into account the needs of disabled students. They must provide disability statements about the facilities available for such students, which should include details such as access, the specialist equipment and counselling available, admission arrangements, and complaints and appeals procedures for disabled students. The Act applies in Northern Ireland with exceptions. There are three main areas where disabilities may have an impact on medical work.

- The doctor's condition may limit/reduce/prevent him/her from performing the job effectively.
- The condition may be made worse by the job or make it unsafe for the doctor to do the job.
- The condition might make the tasks unsafe both for the doctor and for fellow workers or for the patients and the community.

There are many demanding aspects to medical work, and any disability that might impede clinical capability needs to be considered carefully. It may be appropriate for students to have a skills assessment to ensure that they are fit to perform the tasks involved in becoming a doctor. This will focus on what the student can do, rather than what they cannot do. The medical school faculty and occupational health services may be able to offer skills assessment and advice. Deans of medical schools should be able to offer further information and advice. Students may be eligible for financial help, such as the disabled students' allowance. Following a publication by its Disabled Doctors Working Party titled *Meeting the Needs of Doctors with Disabilities*, the BMA launched a service for disabled medical students and doctors. This aims to provide information about aids, facilities, equipment, and financial help. It will also put disabled medical students and doctors in touch with each other. Further information may be obtained from the Medical Education Department, BMA House, Tavistock Square, London WC1H 9JR.

Overseas students

Applicants from outside the UK must apply via UCAS and should follow the instructions in the *UCAS Handbook*. You can get copies of the UCAS information from British Council offices or by writing to UCAS. Many schools and colleges will order supplies for you. The British Council will have information about UK universities and medical schools. It will also be able to guide you on whether your qualifications are recognised in the UK. British Embassies or High Commissions and your own country's education authorities will be able to advise you on grants and scholarships. You should also make contact with your preferred medical schools directly. If you are not studying UK-examined

A-levels, then contact the admissions office at the medical school to check whether your subject choices and qualifications are acceptable. There are growing links between overseas medical schools and UK schools, and you may be able to do some of your studies in the UK even if you don't get a full-time place on the course. If you are applying to medical schools in other countries you might want to enquire about this.

Expansion of places

For the first time in many years the actual number of institutions at which you can study medicine is increasing. In 1999 the government announced an initial increase of 1000 places at medical schools, and further announcements have been made which will continue this expansion. To accommodate the rise in the number of medics, some schools have been allowed to increase their intake, and three new centres of undergraduate medical education have been opened. New centres already open are at Durham (Stockton), Keele and Warwick. These represent joint ventures with existing schools at Newcastle, Manchester, and Leicester, respectively. We have put some information about the courses at these centres alongside the information about the existing course at the partner institute. The majority of the new places have been added to the existing medical degree courses, and those at Durham and Keele will involve periods of study at the new centre as well as at the established one.

New courses specifically for graduate entrants have started at Cambridge, Leicester/Warwick, Oxford and St George's, and more are planned at other schools. Brand new medical schools at the Universities of East Anglia, Exeter and Plymouth (Peninsula Medical School), Brighton and Sussex, and York and Hull are scheduled to take their first students in 2002 and 2003. The new Welsh Assembly is considering how medical student numbers might be increased in Wales. Ideas include a school at Swansea or Bangor.

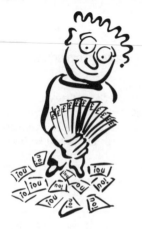

6

Funding your way through

What to expect

Money is an issue close to most students' hearts, and medical students are no exception. Government reforms of the higher education funding system, such as the introduction of tuition fees and the abolition of maintenance grants in 1998, have meant that the issue of debt is one that is affecting many more students than in previous years.

A recent BMA report (*Annual Survey of Medical Students' Finances 2000/2001*) found that the average total debt among final-year students was over £13 000. More than 40% of final-year medical students had debts in excess of £15 000. Although this may seem quite daunting you shouldn't let it put you off studying medicine. Yes, you are likely to be in more debt after graduation than someone who takes a three-year degree course, but this is balanced by excellent future career prospects and good job security. Medical student intake reflects all sectors of society. If you are not supported by wealthy or generous parents **you won't be alone** in being in debt, and it won't be forever. There are currently more jobs than there are doctors in the UK, and this trend looks set to continue for some time, so unemployment after graduation is not really an issue. Most medical graduates pay off their debt within five years of graduation, which helps to explain why bank managers tend to be very welcoming to medics!

Medicine is a four-year course at least and can be as long as six years, so you will have to consider how you will support yourself for that time. The first two years are often the least financially demanding, as a great proportion of your year will be holidays. For many, this allows living at home for half the year and saving some costs; also, you will have plenty of time to earn cash in the holidays, if you want or need to. It gets a little trickier in your clinical years (when you spend more time in hospital): a total annual holiday of six weeks is considered good! During this time you'll have to pay for rent and food for the whole year, and it becomes difficult to find paid work when you have only six weeks off. Some students get part-time jobs during term time, although it is not always easy to fit this in. There are many kinds of expenses involved in studying medicine, and debt is likely to stare you in the face earlier than you might anticipate. Medicine is different from almost any degree course and there are several additional expenses: for example, there will be many expensive books to buy – you could spend at least £150 per year – and medical equipment, such as stethoscopes, can cost around £60. You will also need some smart clothing once you're in hospitals regularly. This is to make you look and feel like part of the medical profession, and to help you gain patient trust.

The financial issue of the moment is the proposed introduction of "**differential fees**", which could be as much as £13 000 per year. Student bodies are opposed to their introduction, as they will discourage people from attending university because they simply cannot afford it. The BMA's Medical Students Committee (MSC) is campaigning vehemently to prevent their institution and to relay this to central government. The government's recent White Paper on Higher Education outlines proposals for funding higher education in the future. More information is available on the BMA website but changes are not likely to come into force for a few years. Please contact individual universities to find out the exact situation – even though they may have no plans to charge additional fees at present, will they expect you to pay if they are introduced halfway through your course?

The obvious question is "How will I pay for all this?". The first port of call for many people will be parents, guardians, or family, who may be able to give you something towards the cost of studying. If they are generous the problem is solved, but if not (which applies to most of us) then there are government loans, bank loans, overdrafts, and many other ways to fund yourself through university.

The type of funding you receive depends on a couple of factors: where you live in the UK and whether you have a previous degree. Funding arrangements for Scottish and graduate students will be discussed later in the chapter.

2002 saw the introduction of the NHS bursary, which means funding arrangements are different depending on which year of the course you are in, but this will be explained in the following sections.

Costs associated with studying medicine

Tuition fees

Since October 1998, students have been required to contribute towards the cost of their education. For 2002/2003 the maximum home students had to pay was £1100 per year. If your family income is below a certain level (approximately £20 500 pa) you will not be expected to pay tuition fees at all. The full amount will only be payable if your parents' residual income is in excess of £30 502. Tuition fees make up a proportion of the cost of your tuition, the rest of which is made up by your Local Education Authority (LEA) in the form of mandatory and discretionary awards.

The BMA's MSC persuaded the government that special consideration needed to be given to medical students because of the length and expense of the course, and the Department of Health agreed to pay tuition fees for medical students from year 5 onwards. This also applies to students doing premedical or intercalated years. This means that you will only pay tuition fees for the first four years of your course.

Living costs

Money for accommodation, food, transport, books, and beer will come from parental contributions, maintenance loans and, invariably, banks. The amount of maintenance loan you will be entitled to will depend on where you study and what year you are in. Loans are administered by the Student Loans Company. Twenty-five per cent of the loan is means tested and will depend largely upon your parents' income. The maximum loan available in 2002/2003 for students outside London was £3905 and for those in London was £4815, with smaller amounts being available to students living at home. Student loan repayments will be paid in instalments after graduation, once your income is over £10 000 per year. For medics, repayments will begin during your first house officer job, which will generally be a few months after finals. There is extra money available for courses that last longer than 30 weeks. In response to campaigns by the MSC, the Department of Health has agreed to provide means-tested non-repayable bursaries for medical students from year 5 onwards, which students will be able to apply for in addition to student loans. Students taking premedical and/or intercalated years will also be able to apply for this from year 5 onwards.

Travelling expenses

Most of the teaching on medical courses takes place on clinical attachments in hospitals and GP surgeries. These can be quite a distance from your main medical school base and travelling expenses can be considerable. It is expected that most students will fund travel expenses out of maintenance loans, although some may be claimed back from your LEA. The rules currently state that you can claim back travelling expenses incurred in attending clinical placements, although the first £265 must be borne by you. The amount you receive will be means tested. You should contact your local LEA to find out the arrangements for claiming expenses, and keep receipts and a record of journeys made to help your claim.

Boosting your funds

High-street bank

In addition to the maintenance loan, a bank overdraft is likely to be required. Surviving at medical school makes this an almost essential part of your finances. Most banks and building societies offer students special terms on bank accounts. These normally include interest-free overdrafts. Keeping your bank manager happy by not exceeding the agreed overdraft limit is good practice, and also helps you avoid penalty charges and punishing interest rates. If you want to extend your overdraft, go and discuss it with the manager face to face. The bank wants your custom because you will have a good job at the end of your university career, and they are experienced at helping students out with money problems. Banks are more likely to be generous and sympathetic with students who keep them informed than those who constantly surprise them. If you need more cash than an overdraft gives you, then you may need a loan. Look around to make sure you have accessed all other sources of funding before you take out a loan, for example hardship funds and charitable funds (see below). Banks can be willing to accept begging letters and IOUs from medics, and many have specially tailored loans of up to £20 000 for medical students.

Remember, though: the debt you incur will have to be paid back regardless. Do not be blasé – heaven forbid that through illness, failure, or other unpredictable acts you do not qualify and are unable to repay your debts. Such instances are rare, but it would be irresponsible for us to overlook these possibilities. Make sure you fully understand the terms of the loan and shop around for the best deal. Don't just go to the bank you have an account with – it won't necessarily offer you the best deal.

Charities

There are literally hundreds of educational trust funds and charities in the UK, many of which support medical students. They tend to be open to mature and graduate students rather than school leavers, but it may be worth trying to find some funding from these sources. General directories of charitable trusts are available in the reference section of most public libraries and some are listed in the Further information section of this book. Spending time searching through the lists and applying for grants may be to your advantage. Many small trusts have bizarre criteria for offering awards, and you may be surprised to find that by meeting the unusual requirements you can get help towards your expenses.

Access funds, hardship funds and hardship loans

Universities receive money from the government to help students in the poorest financial shape. Applications for the money are processed locally and policies on how these funds are distributed vary widely from school to school. It is important to be aware that this money is available.

Work

For the majority of medical undergraduates, working during vacations in the early part of the course is a necessity. As well as casual work in bars and restaurants, many students work as healthcare assistants and medical secretaries. Work can usually be arranged through the teaching hospital or other local hospitals. The experience of working in a hospital environment in a role other than as a medical practitioner can be very valuable. As the course progresses, however, the holidays get shorter as term time extends and periods of elective study intervene, and it then becomes more difficult to find employment for these shorter periods. You might consider taking a part-time job during term. The medical course is undoubtedly challenging and demands a lot of your time in studying, no matter how gifted you are. Because of this, some medical schools discourage students from working during term. They cannot actually prevent you from doing so, but be warned that they may take a dim view. Check out the school's attitude with the medics on open days. Do not let a job get in the way of studies.

A small number of medical students sign up to one of the Armed Forces medical cadet schemes. A "salary" is paid to cadets for two to three years. In return for this support during undergraduate training cadets serve as an officer with, for example, the Royal Army Medical Corps, for a minimum period of duty (normally six years after full qualification). The income cadets receive is very generous compared to other students' incomes, but the quid pro quo is the six-year short service commission. You will continue to practise as a doctor, but the Ministry of Defence will require you to support military initiatives anywhere in the world. Working as a doctor in the Armed Forces can be very rewarding and challenging. It is the advice of the authors of this guide that students who embark on medical cadetships should be committed to a career in the Services after graduation, and not simply addressing the funding of their course. The Forces recruit during the early years of the medical degree course and offer familiarisation visits for interested students. Contact details for each Service are given in the Further information section at the end of the book.

Elective funding

Students who organise themselves well in advance can often get enough funding to pay for some (if not all) of the cost of their elective. You should have a wonderful time wherever you go, but it is so much nicer if you know you haven't paid for it all yourself. Depending on where you want to go and what you will be studying, there are numerous grants, research awards, sponsorships, and bursaries available. Some will be open for all UK students to apply for, and other funds will be distributed locally. Most awards and grants are given in exchange for some sort of project report or research work.

Graduate students

Tuition fees

Fees for graduate students or self-funding students on standard courses will vary from institution to institution (see later). Some charge the standard £1100 per year, whereas others charge more for the preclinical stage of the course and more again for the clinical stage, so it is important to bear this in mind before applying and check with each medical school. Graduates who have received support from public funds for their first degree are not entitled to receive any mandatory or discretionary funding from their LEA and would therefore be liable to pay the full cost of tuition throughout the course. The MSC has been calling on medical schools to limit the amount of fees payable by graduates to the standard £1100, but there is no guarantee of success. In response to campaigns by the MSC, the government has introduced concessions for graduate medical students on the four-year accelerated degree courses being held at Cambridge, St George's, and Leicester/Warwick. Tuition fees are paid by the Department of Health in years 2, 3, and 4 of the course and fees are payable by the students in year 1 only. The MSC is trying to persuade government to extend this scheme to graduate entrants on any medical degree course.

Scottish students studying on an accelerated course in the UK do not receive NHS tuition fee and bursary support in years 2 to 4, and are treated as though they were graduate students on a standard course, that is, means-tested maintenance loans and tuition fees.

Living costs

Graduate medical students are entitled to apply to the Student Loans Company for help with their living costs. The maximum loan available in 2002/2003 for students outside London was £3905 and for those in London it was £4815 – 25% of the loan is means tested and will depend largely upon your personal/spousal income. These figures are revised annually. Graduates on accelerated courses can apply for funding to the NHS bursary scheme in years 2, 3, and 4 of the course. Under-25s are subject to a parental means test if they apply for a bursary, and this limits its availability. The MSC is pressing for this criterion to be relaxed. Graduates on standard courses will be able to apply to the NHS bursary from year 5 onwards.

Scottish students

Arrangements for Scottish students vary according to whether they are studying in Scotland or elsewhere in the UK. The Student Awards Agency for Scotland (SAAS) is the body that deals with student support in Scotland (see Further information).

Tuition fees

Students studying at Scottish universities will not have to make a contribution to tuition fees. The Scottish Executive has set up a graduate endowment scheme whereby graduates will contribute a sum of around £2030 after they have left university (2002/2003 entrant figures). The funds raised will be used to support future students. Repayment of the endowment begins after you start earning more than £10 000 per year (in your house job). The "St Andrew's anomaly", where the preclinical students go on to do clinical studies elsewhere (usually Manchester), and therefore which funding scheme they fit into, is yet to be settled.

Living costs

The living support package you will receive differs according to whether you are classed as a young or a mature student. The Scottish Executive has introduced non-repayable maintenance grants of up to £2050 per year for students from families on low incomes and mature students with children. Maintenance loans from the Student Loans Company are also available.

Scottish students studying elsewhere in the UK

The funding for students studying outside Scotland is quite similar to that of other UK students. Your entitlement to tuition fee support is parental income assessed (up to £1100 for 2002/2003). Where there is a contribution to be deducted from the tuition fee support, the SAAS will pay the remainder.

Living costs support comes from student loans, which are the same as in the rest of the UK. There is an additional "Young Students Outside Scotland Bursary" which is available for students from families with an income below £18 400. Mature students may apply for additional grants towards the cost of childcare.

Support in the fifth year and beyond for Scottish students

All Scottish students, regardless of their place of study, can claim an income-assessed NHS bursary and free tuition. You will also have access to a non-income-assessed student loan, repayable once your income has reached a set level, currently around £10 000 pa.

The final balance ...

Irrespective of your personal circumstances, studying medicine means undertaking a serious financial commitment. In common with many other students you will have to face up to some debt and financial worries. By accepting this reality and planning before you start how your tuition fees, parents' contribution, bank overdraft, student loan and bank loans will fit together over the years, you will come to terms with it better. You can find information about funding in our Further information section. Make sure your acquaintance with debt is on your own terms. Do not avoid dealing with tough money questions and do not adopt a head-in-the-sand approach to your finances. If you anticipate difficulties during the course, take advice from the Students Union welfare services, the university and your bank. Don't leave it too late to take action – there are very few miracle workers, and the people who are there to help are more likely to be helpful if they are given time. This talk of poverty and debt is depressing, but remember these two things.

- Debt is now a fact of life for students, and the vast majority survive and free themselves from its tyranny.
- Medical students are better placed than most to pay off their debts at the end of the day, with excellent employment prospects and job security.

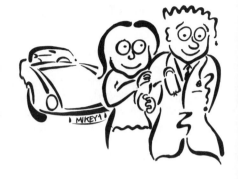

7

Life beyond graduation ...

The preregistration house officer year(s)

Graduating or qualifying from medical school with an MBChB or MBBS does not, in itself, allow you to practise medicine: first you must register with the GMC. Initially, registration with the Council is only provisional, but you can call yourself Doctor. To register fully, newly qualified doctors are required to complete 12 months of paid work as a preregistration house officer (PRHO) or "house officer". This has traditionally consisted of a six-month post in medicine and a six-month post in surgery. However, many hospital trusts, in partnership with the postgraduate deanery, now offer new composite posts which consist of four months in medicine, four in surgery, then a further four in an alternative specialty such as paediatrics, general practice, accident and emergency or psychiatry. The government has recently proposed wide-ranging reform of house officer posts, including extending the PRHO year to a two-year programme which, it claims, will benefit the future career choices of junior doctors.

House officer posts must be approved by the GMC for the experience to count towards full registration. If you complete these posts satisfactorily, you can apply for full GMC registration. Free hospital accommodation is provided for your job because the GMC believes that the right type of experience is only gained if you are resident, so don't worry if your jobs are in parts of the country you didn't choose: there will be accommodation provided. More information about the PRHO year can be found in the BMA document *First House Job*, revised in August 2002.

Applying for PRHO jobs

Most areas operate some sort of matching scheme in the final (or penultimate) year, which is normally coordinated by the postgraduate deanery. A house officer job-matching scheme does what it suggests – it matches prospective house officers to house officer posts. Some schemes are open to medics from any UK medical school, and some are only open to the university's own students. Some only cover the posts in the university teaching hospitals, and some cover all the hospitals in the region. Normally, the school that sends students to a hospital for clinical experience will supply the same hospital with its new house officers, but some schemes include posts that are many miles away. If you are clear that you want to work in a particular part of the country, it might be worth finding out about the matching scheme. However, remember that by the time you graduate the scheme might have changed.

The advantage of matching schemes is that some of the work needed to find a job is done for you and you will only be placed in university-approved jobs. The downside is that some schemes give you little notice of where your first house job will be or leave you feeling alienated from the process. Some medical schools produce too few graduates to fill all the regional posts and some produce too many, but for the foreseeable future medics have good prospects of getting work. If you cannot get a house job in the particular town or city you would like to work in, don't worry. During the training years you can apply for jobs elsewhere in the country (and abroad). Hospitals in Australasia, for example, recruit UK doctors for short-term posts.

The BMA also provides an interactive house jobs guide for members on its website. The guide has information from hospital trusts as well as from junior doctors actually working in the trust. Having a look at this guide when you reach your fourth and fifth years of medical school may prove helpful.

Life as the house dog

The year as a house surgeon and physician is often the toughest in a medical career. There is much to do and learn, and sometimes providing a service to patients and your employer is at the cost of your continuing education. You are well and truly at the bottom of the medical hierarchy and demands from your patients, your colleagues, and your bosses can be overpowering. Hours of work are long (50+ per week), despite the European Working Time Directive. Working intensively at night or weekends (on call) can be exhausting. As a house officer you will be responsible for taking histories from new patients, organising tests, following up consultants' instructions, and helping at outpatient clinics and with theatre sessions. However, there are controls and ways of reducing the strains upon you. There will probably be times when you are fed up and may want to quit medicine. Some do, but the vast majority stay on. You will become more confident, more able to cope, and the work will eventually become more interesting (and challenging).

Beyond the house officer year

After the house officer year your career can begin to follow the path you want it to. For most junior doctors this is initially in senior house officer posts through general professional or basic specialist training and, later, in specialist or GP registrar posts. If you have a strong idea about what specialty you want to practise in or you know you want to become a GP, then you can begin to take the appropriate path through the **training grades**. Don't worry if you don't know which branch of medicine you want to be in now or even, for that matter, during the first few years after graduation. Many SHOs don't decide on their final career until well into their postgraduate training. The two main areas of practice are general practice and hospital (specialty) medicine. In response to growing dissatisfaction with SHO job structure and training, in August 2002 the government released a consultation document entitled *Unfinished Business* setting out their strategy for the reform of the SHO grade over the next few years, and including a plan to make the PRHO year a two-year foundation programme. The BMA did not support this proposal because of the lack of specific information regarding what the second year would entail, and is awaiting further clarification on how the proposal would dovetail with education and professional outcomes. Should the proposal be introduced, the BMA would seek to negotiate an above-average pay award for PRHOs as a way of addressing stress and anxiety.

A career in general practice

General practice is changing significantly, but currently the majority of GPs are called principals. This means they are self-employed doctors who provide general medical services to patients for a health authority. They usually work in groups, which are small business partnerships. The most common route to becoming a principal is to do three years' training as a GP registrar. This is divided into two years of hospital posts (in specialties such as general medicine, general surgery, A&E, obstetrics, geriatrics or psychiatry) and one year working as a "trainee" in general practice. Most doctors training to enter general practice follow vocational training schemes in which the particular posts they will rotate through are preplanned from the outset. By the time the most recent entrants to medical school graduate, it is anticipated that a greater percentage of GPs will be employees rather than independent contractors.

A career in hospital medicine

In order to become a hospital consultant, junior doctors normally rotate through two or three years of SHO jobs in medical or surgical specialties. After this, and once their choice of specialty is clear, they spend between four and five years studying in registrar posts. There are specialist registrar "rotations" which allow a doctor to prearrange three or four years of training in different hospital posts. When this training is completed satisfactorily, a Certificate of Completion of Specialist Training (CCST) is issued and the doctor can apply for consultant posts.

Other career paths

General practice and hospital posts provide the greatest number of jobs for doctors in the health service, but there are many other career paths. Many doctors work in public health medicine, as medical academics, as researchers for pharmaceutical companies, for the Armed Forces, and in private medicine. A great strength of practising as a doctor is the range of experience you can find in work. Flexible training is becoming more common and part-time posts are numerous. Many doctors have more than one string to their bow and it is not uncommon, for example, for a doctor to mix private work or part-time work with their main NHS job. Putting together a portfolio career as a doctor is possible. A consultant might add some medical journalism and legal work in courts as an expert witness to their weekly duties as a hospital specialist; a director of public health might do voluntary medical work with a charity; or a GP might work part time with a local rugby club. The following diagram shows a simplified path of career options in medicine for doctors in the UK.

Medical career structure[1] (reproduced with permission from *Medical Careers: A General Guide*, BMA, 1990)

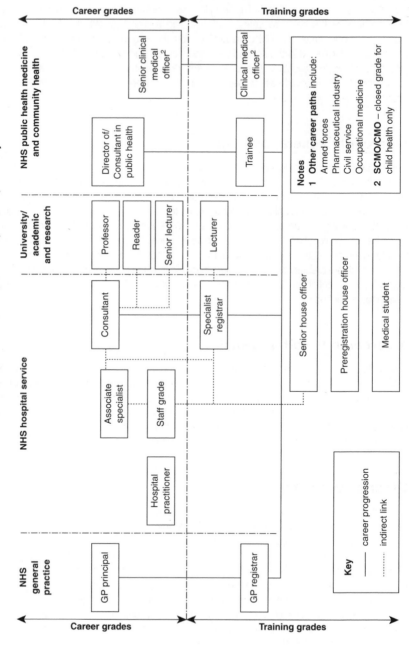

Career grades

Training grades

NHS general practice

GP principal

GP registrar

NHS hospital service

Hospital practitioner

Associate specialist

Staff grade

Consultant

Specialist registrar

Senior house officer

Preregistration house officer

Medical student

University/academic and research

Professor

Reader

Senior lecturer

Lecturer

NHS public health medicine and community health

Senior clinical medical officer[2]

Director of/Consultant in public health

Clinical medical officer[2]

Trainee

Notes

1 **Other career paths** include:
Armed forces
Pharmaceutical industry
Civil service
Occupational medicine

2 **SCMO/CMO** – closed grade for child health only

Key

—— career progression

······ indirect link

Career grades

Training grades

Continuing medical education

Doctors must continue to study after they graduate and they are expected to keep their skills and knowledge up to date. This is a requirement from the GMC. The Council is introducing a system of formal reassessment for all doctors on its register – *revalidation*. Many skills and much knowledge will be acquired "on the job", but most career paths require some formal qualifications and exams will have to be passed. The Royal Colleges are responsible for medical education, and for many specialties you will need to pass membership exams to get on in your career. In other specialties diplomas and Royal College membership exams are encouraged to supplement the minimum standards required. It was partly to encourage a positive attitude towards lifelong learning that the GMC introduced changes to the undergraduate curriculum that foster learning skills and self-motivation.

Part 2
A–Z of UK medical schools

Aberdeen

Key facts	Aberdeen
Course length	5 years
Total number of medical undergraduates	903
Applicants in 2002	1214
Interviews given in 2002	All students who are in the UK during the year of application are expected to attend for interview. A number of overseas applicants are interviewed in their home country by university representatives
Places available in 2002	175
Places available in 2003	175
Entrance requirements	ABB
Mandatory subjects	None, although chemistry is highly desirable
Male:female ratio	49:51
Premed course	No
Graduate course offered	Yes Fast track. Graduates in appropriate disciplines can enter direct into Phase II

The grey colour and cold temperature of the "granite city" bear no relation to the warm and friendly atmosphere and busy social life that is Aberdeen. The age of the medical school is not reflected in the curriculum – a new integrated systems-based course which exploits technology to its full advantage, something that was commented on when Aberdeen was rated as excellent in a recent appraisal. Everything at the medical school/teaching hospital is on a single site (20–25 minutes' walk from main campus), so you can go straight from lectures to wards. Aberdeen medics tend to work hard, play hard, and make the most out of being a large and distinct department within a university.

Education

The five years are split into four phases: fundamentals of medical science; principles of clinical medicine; specialist clinical practice; and professional practice. A core syllabus focusing on integrated systems for the whole class is counterbalanced with special study modules (SSMs) for the individual. Students must complete each phase before passing on to the next. The first graduates from the new course qualified in summer 2000. Students must adopt a proactive approach, and self-motivation is an important requirement. Although the course is predominantly lecture based, there are problem-based and tutorial-based learning sessions. Some of the course is taught through self-study packages. There is a formal staff/student committee that meets regularly and a clinical staff/student committee that meets every five weeks to discuss the course. Different students attend each time to give a wider viewpoint.

Teaching

Aberdeen received a very high rating in the last Scottish Higher Education Funding Council Teaching Quality assessment. Problem-based teaching is partly replacing the traditional didactic approach and students experience many different learning environments, such as general practice, specialist hospital wards, lecture theatres, tutorial groups and the Clinical Skills Centre. Anatomy is taught via dissection. Computer-assisted learning is integrated within each phase of medical training, supplementing the compulsory ward teaching and tutorials.

Assessment

Assessment is both continual and exam based (written and clinical), with vivas for distinction and pass-fail candidates. There is no compulsory use of animals or animal material in practicals. Should you fail a degree assessment, there are three more chances by way of two vivas and a further written exam. Students are supported and encouraged should this occur.

Intercalated degrees

About one in five students does an intercalated degree (BSc) after year 3. You must have passed all your exams and not repeated a year to be considered. All intercalated students follow a core syllabus as part of their year, followed by a research project – which can be chosen by the student. Many of these projects offer a chance to participate in clinical research, and some students have had their work published in medical journals.

Special study modules and electives

All of the four phases of the course include special study modules. The final phase SSM is non-medical, offering the opportunity to study subjects such as Spanish, history of medicine, music or sign language. During the final phase, students have a seven-week elective period which can be spent abroad, almost anywhere in the world. This includes a short research project, which contributes towards your final degree. It is not a holiday!

Facilities

Library   Library facilities are good (open 8.45 am–10 pm Monday to Thursday; 8.45 am–8 pm Friday; 9 am–10 pm Saturday; 1 pm–10 pm Sunday). Texts and journals are plentiful, as is access to Medline. Photocopying costs approx 3p/sheet, and printing 5p/sheet.

Computers   There are many computers available, with free internet and email, although at times a shortage of printers. There are excellent computer-assisted learning packages for a variety of subjects, as well as practice exam questions. Many lecture presentations are available on the internet. There is 24-hour access to computer laboratories on the university campus and at the medical school.

Clinical skills   The clinical skills laboratory sited in the hospital grounds is equipped with up-to-date medical technology. It is used for teaching clinical skills and procedures to all medical students and junior doctors, with timetabled access and "drop-in" sessions run by senior specialists (eye examination by an ophthalmologist, for example). These include examination skills, use of equipment, communication skills (interviewing simulated patients), and many practical procedures, e.g. IV access, suturing, catheterisation, defibrillation, etc. A "Harvey" cardiology patient simulator is now used to teach all students from second year upwards.

Welfare

Student support

There are regular staff–student liaison meetings, excellent relationships with lecturers, and the Dean is very approachable. There is a large support network should things go wrong, including academic tutors, individual advisors ("Regent Scheme"), trained counselling staff at the university, and the usual main university NUS welfare support.

Accommodation

University flats and halls accommodation are readily available for all years of study, although most people move into private accommodation after their first year. Private accommodation is in high demand and can be expensive.

Placements

Everything at the medical school is at the Foresterhill Hospital site, so you can go straight from lectures to the wards. During the final two years you study on attachment to hospitals in either Inverness, Fort William, or Elgin for 5–10 weeks. Placements in Shetland and Stornoway, introduced in 2001, were oversubscribed with volunteers. Moreover, GP attachments are now available throughout Scotland. Free accommodation is provided, as is travel at the beginning and end of the attachments. Most of the GP placements are in rural general practice.

Studying at one of the largest teaching hospitals in Europe allows Aberdeen medical students to experience all specialties on a single site. A new children's hospital is due to open on site in 2003. The learning environment is relaxed and friendly, with the medical staff rewarding you with the help you need as long as you put in the effort. Also, getting written finals over with at the end of the fourth year leaves time to earn up to £160 a week working as a student locum. Students on placements away from Aberdeen enjoy excellent teaching, social life, and free accommodation close to the hospital. The newly introduced "island" attachments involve one-to-one teaching from a consultant: excellent experience, especially if you are a budding surgeon. However, some students might find these placements a bit too isolated.

Sports and social

City life

The city centre is compact and lively, with most pubs/clubs within 10 minutes' walk of each other and 20 minutes' walk from most student halls. Aberdeen is a prosperous town. The revenue brought in by the oil industry is apparent when looking at the excellent provision of shops, pubs and other services. Because of this Aberdeen can be expensive to live in. Glasgow and Edinburgh are both easily accessible, and Aberdeen has excellent travel links.

City and surrounds Just a short journey from the buzzing centre is the beach, with roller coasters, an ice-rink, and a new cinema. In the other direction are the hills and the outdoors: excellent for walking, climbing, winter and water sports. The northerly location means the climate can be very cold and, although there are road, rail, and air links, Aberdeen is a considerable distance from anywhere else. People from far away (UK and overseas) can get a bit homesick and find Aberdonians more hostile than they actually are – but the strong friendships you will make in Aberdeen will help you through this.

Uni life

As the medical school is isolated from other parts of the university, medics need to make a bit of an effort to meet non-medical students, but the first year is normally spent in halls and this gives students an opportunity to meet others outside medicine. Most student social life tends to revolve around drinking! The union runs many organised events and the Medical Society holds functions every two to three weeks and hosts a very popular annual ball. University societies are numerous and healthy, covering a wide range of interests: sporting, dramatic, photography, musical, outdoor, university Armed Forces units (army, navy, and RAF), intellectual, malt whisky appreciation, etc. The medical school has a few societies of its own, and the annual medical revue is well supported and popular.

Sports life

The Aberdeen Medical Students Society (MedSoc) has its own rugby, football, cricket, and hockey teams, which compete against the other Scottish medical schools. MedSoc members can join an exclusive gym in town for a discounted fee of £100 per year. The main university offers a wide range of sports as varied as gliding, underwater hockey, and archery, as well as regulars such as rugby, hockey, and football. Members of all levels are given a warm welcome. There are no specific medical school facilities, but the university offers an inexpensive gym, pool, and tennis facilities, among others.

Additional application information

Average A-level requirements	• ABB – Chemistry is highly desirable, plus at least one from biology, mathematics or physics and one other
Average Scottish Higher requirements	• Five Highers at AAAAB obtained at a single sitting. Chemistry is highly desirable, plus two from biology/human biology, mathematics and physics. Applicants only attempting four Highers owing to school policy or personal difficulties are normally required to achieve AAAA at the first sitting
Make-up of interview panel	• Two Admissions Selectors – with at least one clinician
Months in which interviews are held	• November to March
Proportion of overseas students	• 7%
Proportion of mature students	• Approximately 14%
Faculty's view of students taking a gap year	• Approved, provided the applicant has a plan for the year
Proportion of students taking intercalated degrees	• Approximately 20%
Possibility of direct entrance to clinical phase	• Not impossible, but applicants would need strong support from their current Dean. Approximately 15 places available in second year for graduate entrants
Fees for graduates	• See Chapter 6
Fees for overseas students	• £9480 pa (preclinical) and £18 000 pa (clinical)
Assistance for elective funding	• Some funds and awards available on merit
Assistance for travel to attachments	• Minibus service/one return journey
Access and hardship funds	• Access bursaries and mature student bursaries. University hardship funds available
Weekly rent	• Halls £41–£86 Private £45–£60
Pint of lager	• Union bar £1.60 City centre pub £2.20
Cinema	• £3.00
Nightclub	• Free–£10

Great things about Aberdeen

- Friendly small school, with teaching hospital and medical school buildings within a single site.
- Excellent student social life, with civilised licensing laws (late opening).
- Easy access to the great outdoors (beach and mountains a very short distance away; skiing 45 minutes away; sailing locally).
- Patient contact from the first term of your first year!
- New clinical skills centre with lots of great teaching equipment and online resources.

Bad things about Aberdeen

- No dedicated medics social centre on site.
- Cold in the winter.
- Travelling from Aberdeen often involves a long journey and living far away from home.
- Geographically isolated from the rest of the university, which means the majority of your student friends are medics. This is not helped by the different timings of exams and holidays.
- It's cold most of the rest of the year too!

Further information

Medical Faculty Office (Admissions)
Polwarth Building
Medical School
Foresterhill
Aberdeen AB25 2ZD
Tel: 01224 554975
Fax: 01224 840708
Email: f.a.galloway@abdn.ac.uk
Web: http://www.abdn.ac.uk/medicine/prospective-students

Belfast

Key facts	Belfast
Course length	5 years
Total number of medical undergraduates	904
Applicants in 2002	551
Interviews given in 2002	7%
Places available in 2002	181
Places available in 2003	180
Entrance requirements	AAB + A (AS) although under review for 2004
Mandatory subjects	Chemistry + another science. Biology at least to AS
Male:female ratio	34:66
Premed course	Yes – limited number of places for non-A-level students
Graduate course offered	No

Queen's University of Belfast provides a relaxed and informal integrated medical course. Ninety per cent of the students come from Ireland (both north and south), and a strong emphasis is placed on social life and enjoyment. The school also sits in a perfect position to access Belfast's nightlife, arguably the best in the UK. Queen's is the only medical school where it is not illegal to enjoy a good night's craic!! Discussions are taking place to increase the size of the medical school, with more undergraduate places. However, as yet there have been no plans to implement a graduate accelerated course.

Education

A traditional preclinical/clinical divide is less evident on the new course, and teaching combines a problem-based approach with more traditional lectures from the first year. Clinical skills are taught from year 1 in hospitals, in general practice, and in a clinical skills centre. Each year is divided into two semesters, and the trend is for year groups to be divided into smaller groups for teaching. In years 1 and 2 students learn the basic science of medicine with an integrated systems approach. The sociological and psychological aspects of medical practice are emphasised and special study modules are taken. In year 3 the systems are taught again, but with an emphasis on mechanisms of disease. More time is spent in hospital attachments at this stage, and year 4 students spend all their time on the wards in hospital attachments or in general practice. The final year is a consolidation process with no new subjects.

Teaching

Teaching in years 1 and 2 consists of lectures, tutorials, laboratory practicals and meeting patients, both on the wards and in general practice. There is a mixture of demonstration, dissection, and prosection for teaching, and animal tissue is used in physiology. During years 1 and 2 only half a day a week is spent on the wards. In year 3 blocks of specialty-based integrated teaching are supplemented by pathology laboratory classes. Teaching is very much self-directed, with the clinical aspects being taught on the wards. Years 4 and 5 are completely ward based. Computers and clinical skills are used for training throughout the course. Ward group sizes in teaching hospitals tend to vary, but efforts are made to keep the numbers as small as possible to benefit both the patients and the students. The friendliness of the staff and their willingness to teach varies from ward to ward. Most, however, are willing to help in true Northern Ireland fashion.

Assessment

In the first three years examinations are at the end of each semester, whereas those in year 4 are at the end of each eight-week block. Resit examinations start in the second week of August and last for a week or two. Most try to give exams their best so as to maximise the holiday period. Procedure cards need to be completed as part of A&E medicine, anaesthetics, fractures, and obstetrics and gynaecology. Final examinations take place in two parts. The written examinations take place in September at the start of the final year, and the clinical examinations are held at the end of the final year. During the final year the overseas elective, a clinical project, refresher clinical placements, and a clinical apprenticeship are completed.

Intercalated degrees

Between 5% and 10% of students take a BSc during their course, usually after years 2 or 3. Science degrees are available in anatomy, biochemistry, physiology, microbiology, pharmacology, and medical genetics. It is possible to study degree subjects that are not available at Queen's by making arrangements with another institution. Approval for this, however, has to be sought from the Dean. If there is competition for places, previous results in the respective subject will determine entry. Students from Northern Ireland may be eligible for Local Education Authority (LEA) or bursary funding for the year.

Special study modules and electives

During the summer vacation between years 3 and 4 students have the option to arrange elective pupilships for a period of four to six weeks at a hospital in the UK. This is optional and the student takes responsibility for organisation. In the final year students are encouraged to spend their elective period overseas. Students must also carry out a six-week clinical project, either overseas or at Queen's, followed by the production of a project report of between 7000 and 10 000 words.

Facilities

Library   There are two medical libraries, the largest in the Royal Victoria Hospital (RVH) and a smaller one in the Belfast City Hospital (BCH). They both have online catalogues, with access to networked journals, Medline, and other databases. They close at 9.30 pm on weekdays and 12.30 pm on Saturdays. Study space is available at the Belfast City Hospital and at the Medical Biology Centre (MBC) outside the library opening hours.

Computers   There are eight computer centres with a total of 523 PCs, for use by all students. Their opening hours vary, but at least one centre is available between 8 am and 12 midnight. Some also open on a 24-hour basis near the exams.

Clinical skills   A new clinical skills laboratory centre was opened in 1996. This is an essential resource for the new course. Facilities are fantastic and they provide a great opportunity to practise clinical skills.

Welfare

Student support

Each medical student is allocated to a consultant, known as their Faculty Tutor, whose role is to help with any problems. Staff in the faculty office are friendly and approachable, as is the current Dean. The Students' Union also has a small counselling service. Rails, ramps, and lifts are available in many areas for disabled access. A recent minding scheme has been started (called MAFIA) whereby each student is allocated a "godfather" who looks after the personal aspects of student life. A key feature of Queen's is that the different year groups mix well.

Accommodation

There are places in university halls for every student who wants one. The rooms tend to be warm and comfortable, with good food but thin walls. Catered rooms cost between £50 and £65 per week and self-catering rooms £45–61.50 per week, inclusive of heat and light. They are about half a mile from the university. Biggart House is on the RVH site, which is very convenient for getting to ward rounds early but necessitates some transport (such as a taxi) to get to the main student area at night. For your isolation you pay £140 per month including electricity (but no meals). Private accommodation costs from £100 to £150 per month, depending on the position and quality.

Placements

In years 1 and 2 most of the teaching takes place on campus in the MBC and the BCH beside it. These are about a 15-20-minute walk from the halls of residence. Other lectures and clinical work take place at the RVH, a 35–40-minute walk from the halls. However, a free bus runs from the BCH to the RVH every 15 minutes. Students from year 3 onwards receive teaching in the RVH, and clinical attachments may be throughout the Province. The Royal Victoria recently underwent renovation, the result of which is a brand new hospital, with great teaching facilities. In addition, from year 3 onwards hospitals and GP practices outside central Belfast are used. Hospital and GP accommodation is free, and the furthest one might travel would be about 80 miles from Belfast.

Sports and social

City life

Despite being the capital of the Province, Belfast is more like a provincial city: small, lively, and not overwhelming. Everything you need as a student is within walking distance, and the centre of Belfast is only a mile away from the university and medical school. There is a good range of pubs, cafes, clubs, and cinemas (including a two-screen "arthouse" cinema). There are theatres, museums, and galleries, and most venues offer student discounts and concessions. Despite its reputation, Belfast in general, and the university area in particular, is a relatively safe place to live. Ninety per cent of students are from Northern Ireland, with 1–2% from the rest of the UK and the rest from overseas. Medical social life focuses around the Belfast Medical Students' Association (BMSA), which runs a wide-ranging programme of events.

Although you may have your hands full coping with what Belfast has to offer, it is easy to travel further afield. Dublin is just over two hours away by train, and it is a must to visit the Giant's Causeway, the Mourne Mountains and the Fermanagh Lakes, all of which are within 1½ hours of Belfast.

Uni life

The BMSA is the oldest and largest student society in the university. Every year the BMSA runs a freshers' three-legged pub crawl, a mystery tour, a fancy dress party, the annual faculty ball, a staff–student dinner, and regular discos which are attended by all years. The fourth year runs its own annual revue – tasteless but entertaining – and a medical charity called SWOT, which raises money by organising blood pressure clinics, street collections, a fashion show (with local TV celebrities), and pub quizzes. Queen's also has an active MedSIN group. The Students' Union has three bars and runs regular discos, balls, and concerts. The Union has undergone a recent revamp and is modern, bright, and friendly. Like most universities, there is likely to be a society for whatever you want to do.

Sports life

There is a men's medics rugby team (the Spiros), which has an annual tour, a football team, and a ski club which pays visits to the Belfast artificial slope. There are many sports clubs at Queen's, most of which compete in the Province's leagues. Near the university there are playing fields, tennis courts, and a boat club. The Queen's Physical Education Centre has everything you need to keep fit. It is beside the university, well equipped, and costs 70p to get in if you are a student.

Great things about Queen's

- An updated curriculum in which students gain clinical experience beginning in year 1 with small group teaching.
- Queen's has an international reputation for trauma care, cardiology, and ophthalmology.
- Belfast is compact as a capital city but has everything you need.
- The social life – fortnightly events are organised by Belfast Medical Students Association (BMSA). Interyear relations are good.
- Relaxed and informal atmosphere.

Bad things about Queen's

- The weather – there is no danger of students blowing their allowance on suntan lotion.
- The weekends tend to be quiet. Many students go home at the weekend, particularly in the first year.
- The siting of the main medical library means that at night students can only get to it by car.
- The ready availability of the "Ulster Fry" pushes your waistband.
- The high number of students on some attachments.

Additional application information

Average A-level requirements	• A-level chemistry at grade A plus at least one other A-level from biology, maths or physics. Biology must be offered at AS-level if not at A-level
Average Scottish Higher requirements	• Considered individually
Make-up of interview panel	• Three (Assistant Head of School of Medicine and two members of academic staff)
Months in which interviews are held	• February
Proportion of overseas students	• 7%
Proportion of mature students	• 5%
Faculty's view of students taking a gap year	• No problem, although students should explain reasons for gap year in personal statement
Proportion of students taking intercalated degrees	• 5–15%
Possibility of direct entrance to clinical phase	• Transfers generally not accepted. There is a formal partnership with the International Medical College in Kuala Lumpur
Fees for graduates	• £1100
Fees for overseas students	• £9865 pa (preclinical) and £18 180 pa (clinical)
Assistance for elective funding	• Vacation grant scheme and faculty bequests are available
Assistance for travel to attachments	• Available through the Education and Library Boards for students entitled to a grant
Access and hardship funds	• Some university funds and bequests are available but amounts are small
Weekly rent	• Halls: Single room catered £65 Single room self-catered £54.50 (£64.50 en suite) Private £35–£50
Pint of lager	• Union bar £1.60 City centre pub £2.00
Cinema	• £2.50–£4
Nightclub	• £2–£10

Further information

Admissions Officer
The Queen's University of Belfast
University Road
Belfast BT7 1NN
Tel: 02890 335081
Fax: 02890 247895
Email: admissions@qub.ac.uk
Web: http://www.qub.ac.uk

Dean's Office
Tel: 02890 245133 ext. 3477
Fax: 02890 330571

Open days: September

Birmingham

Key facts	Birmingham
Course length	5 years
Total number of medical undergraduates	1195
Applicants in 2002	2097
Interviews given in 2002	c. 33%
Places available in 2002	340
Places available in 2003	332
Entrance requirements	AAB
Mandatory subjects	Chemistry (biology to AS)
Male:female ratio	45:55
Premed course	No
Graduate course offered	Yes 4-year fast track

Birmingham Medical School can be found on the northwest edge of the main University of Birmingham campus, just a few miles from the city centre. We are a large provincial medical school, with a huge diversity of students. We have a well-established modern course, with clinical experience introduced from the second week of study. The admissions tutors strongly believe that doctors should be well-rounded individuals and not just dedicated bookworms, and this is reflected in the mix of students and the lively social scene at the medical school, from sport, drama, and politics to partying. From the first week as freshers, students at Birmingham can expect to work hard and play hard until their final-year dinner, held the week before graduation.

Education

The first two years follow a systems-based approach, with regular patient contact in general practice beginning within a few weeks of starting the course. Full-time hospital teaching commences in the third year in both medicine and surgery. Pathology and epidemiology are also taught during this year. Years 4 and 5 involve rotation through specialties such as paediatrics, oncology and orthopaedics, in addition to senior medicine and surgery. Students on the graduate entry course (see Chapter 4), which starts in September 2003, will study the basic sciences in their first year. In their second year they will study a course similar to the standard third year, and will be fully integrated with the rest of the medics for their third and fourth years.

Teaching

Preclinical teaching involves lectures and follow-up tutorials incorporating problem-based learning exercises. There is no dissection at Birmingham, but we have excellent plastinated models to work with in a specially designed laboratory. Histology teaching is all done by video and accompanied by colour course booklets – there is no straining down microscopes for Birmingham medics! Hospital teaching combines bedside teaching, observation, and participation in clinics and procedures.

Assessment

Modules are examined after Christmas and in the summer term by MCQs and short and long answer papers. Some in-course assessment is a feature of most modules. Students are expected to pass every module in order to proceed to the next year. You will also have to pass a practical exam in basic life support during your first year. Viva examinations may be held for borderline pass or Honours candidates. Clinical subjects are examined by MCQ and OSCE.

Intercalated degrees

An increasing number of students at Birmingham are choosing to intercalate, typically after years 2 or 3. Students spend a year studying for an Honours BMedSc. This can be in the biological sciences, such as physiology, pharmacology, neuroscience, or pathology, and involves a laboratory-based research project (and a chance to publish!). Alternatively, you can do an integrated health science, such as public health, ethics and law, behavioural science, or history of medicine. History of medicine is particularly popular and we have an internationally renowned unit based in the medical school.

Special study modules and electives

Eight SSMs are completed during the course. There is a choice of many topics, with new ones starting all the time, which generally become more clinical and self-directed as the course progresses. Electives are taken at the end of the fourth year, with an opportunity to travel anywhere in the world (some bursaries/grants are available, but many students have to find some funding themselves). This normally lasts two months.

Facilities

Library The library is conveniently situated within the medical school and has an extensive range of medical textbooks and journals. It has plenty of quiet study areas and computer facilities with access to Medline, the internet, and library catalogues. It also has extensive photocopying facilities. During term time it is open from 8.45 am to 9 pm Monday–Thursday, until 7 pm on Fridays, and from 10 am to 6 pm at weekends.

Computers   The computer cluster is very futuristic – a vision in blue and steel! There is a mixture of Apple Macs and iMacs (about 100) on the east side, and about 75 PCs on the west side. The computer cluster is open 24 hours, and you are automatically credited with 1000 free laser print credits. Every computer is online and allows full access to computer-assisted learning packages that supplement the course. Computer facilities are also available in general practices, teaching hospitals, and some of the district general hospitals (DGH) that host student teaching.

Welfare

Student support

The pastoral care at Birmingham, from a network of approachable student tutors, is excellent. There is also an effective student-run Curriculum and Welfare Committee that is respected by staff. Students are placed into families, with three to four students from each year group. A social event is held each term by the tutor group, meaning that you will always know a few people in other years.

Accommodation

Accepting a conditional offer from Birmingham guarantees a place in university hall/flats. All university accommodation is within two to three miles of the campus and most is within walking distance. The Vale is a complex of several halls and flats and has the greatest overall capacity. The style of accommodation ranges from large traditional halls to flats with en-suite bathrooms. All halls have good security and excellent committees and social events. There is an excess of private rented accommodation available at reasonable prices in Selly Oak, a Mecca for students and just minutes away from campus. Selly Park, Harborne, and even Edgbaston (which is, in parts, very posh) are also very popular.

Placements

Situated in the suburb of Edgbaston, the university is just a couple of miles from the city centre. The medical school (which adjoins the Queen Elizabeth teaching hospital) is found at the west end of a refreshingly spacious and green campus. It has benefited from the recent refurbishment and upgrading of lecture theatres, tutorial rooms, computer facilities, and student common rooms. The canteen is currently undergoing refurbishment, and should be reopening in the summer of 2003.

There are four large teaching hospitals in the city of Birmingham, as well as specialist hospitals and numerous DGHs. Medics at Birmingham will have very few long-term attachments outside the West Midlands, and the majority of placements are within commuting distance of student accommodation. Help can be provided for travel costs once you are in your clinical years.

During years 1–4, groups of four students attend a general practice once every fortnight. This offers a valuable early introduction to patient contact and clinical skills. The family attachment scheme is another community-based project that takes place in the second year. From the third year onwards, students attend hospital placements full time for most of the year, with occasional teaching sessions in the medical school.

Sports and social

City life

Birmingham is a cosmopolitan city. All the big-name stores and designer shops can be found in the city centre, as well as food to please every palate. Birmingham boasts a vibrant nightlife, ranging from the quintessential student night to jazz clubs and trendy bars. There are plenty of theatres, and the national indoor arena, NEC and Symphony Hall regularly play host to major international acts and are literally on our doorstep! The city and surrounding area are well served by public transport. There is in fact a train station just next to the medical school that connects to Birmingham New Street station, and from there to just about anywhere. Birmingham International Airport is also accessible directly by train. More rural locations, such as the Malverns, Stratford upon Avon, and the Black Country, are all easily reached.

Uni life

Not only is medicine the largest faculty in the university, but related courses such as medical science, physiotherapy, dentistry, and nursing are also based in and around the medical school. There is considerable social integration between all these students and between different year groups. An enthusiastic medical society and final-year dinner committee ensure there is always something happening, and a good time is had by all. As the medical school is located on campus, medics can easily retain involvement in university activities and social events and thus experience the best of both worlds.

A very active medical society and final-year dinner committee take care of the social side of medic life. This includes the renowned freshers' conference, pub crawls, wine tasting, curry quizzes, theatre trips, ski trips, and a post-exam annual camping extravaganza to the Gower. Calendar events held in the medical school include the musical, revue, and final-year fashion show. There is a huge annual medics ball, as well as a summer ball and sports dinners. Many events are held in city centre venues, which are easily accessible by public transport and cheap for a taxi home. The medical school magazine, QMM, was revived a few years ago and affords an opportunity to put pen to paper. There is an active surgical society for those people who think they might be budding surgeons, and MedSIN and Marrow can be found making a difference to the lives of others. The Birmingham University Guild of Students (BUGS) houses the usual complement of bars, clubs, and pool tables, as well as a society for every imaginable interest, from Rag committees to cocktail parties!

Sports life

The university has an excellent reputation for sport. The athletics union runs an impressive range of different sporting clubs. The medics also run large clubs for hockey, rugby, football, netball, cricket, tennis, and basketball. Medics rugby, hockey, and netball teams have all been national medical school champions in recent years. The clubs are friendly and well supported (especially in post-game celebrations) and cater for all ranges of ability, from absolute beginners to international players.

Great things about Birmingham

- Fully integrated new course with early clinical experience keeps your interest levels up.
- Excellent relations between years and with other degree students.
- IT facilities and support are excellent.
- Numerous PRHO jobs available in the region.
- Good range of hospitals used during attachments.

Bad things about Birmingham

- Having to do proper research during the elective (spoiling the holiday).
- The eternal traffic jam on the Bristol Road and M6.
- The wait for exam results, particularly in early years, can be rather long.
- The security guards are very diligent, so if you forget your ID card they won't let you into the medical school.
- Expensive and unvaried food at the medical school canteen.

Additional application information	
Average A-level requirements	• Grades AA in chemistry and one of biology, maths or physics. Biology to AS-level if not A-level
Average Scottish Higher requirements	• AAAAB in chemistry, biology, physics, maths and English and 2 CSYS (any except general studies)
Make-up of interview panel	• Admissions Tutor, two staff and clinical student
Months in which interviews are held	• October–April
Proportion of overseas students	• 10%
Proportion of mature students	• 3%
Faculty's view of students taking a gap year	• No problem provided there are plans to use the year constructively
Proportion of students taking intercalated degrees	• 15–20%
Possibility of direct entrance to clinical phase	• No
Fees for graduates	• £1100 per year. LEA pays year 1. Years 2, 3, and 4 paid by NHS
Fees for overseas students	• £9300 pa (preclinical) and £17 600 pa (clinical)
Assistance for elective funding	• Some competitive bursaries are available
Assistance for travel to attachments	• Yes (clinical years only)
Access and hardship funds	• Some grants and bursaries are available
Weekly rent	• Halls £54–£119 Private £50
Pint of lager	• Union bar £1.60 City centre pub £1.90
Cinema	• £2.50–£4
Nightclub	• £2–£10

Further information

Professor C J Lote
Admissions Officer/Tutor
Medical School
University of Birmingham
Edgbaston
Birmingham B15 2TT
Tel: 0121 414 6888
Fax: 0121 414 7159
Email: c.j.lote@bham.ac.uk, admissions@bham.ac.uk
Prospectus requests: prospectus@bham.ac.uk
Web: http://www.medweb.bham.ac.uk

Open days: April and September

Brighton and Sussex (opening in 2003)

Key facts	Brighton
Course length	5 years
Total number of medical undergraduates	640 (proposed)
Applicants in 2002	–
Interviews given in 2002	–
Places available in 2002	–
Places available in 2003	128
Entrance requirements	ABB
Mandatory subjects	Biology or chemistry A-level (both to AS-level)
Male:female ratio	–
Premed course	No
Graduate course	No

Opening in 2003

The Universities of Brighton and Sussex were successful in their bid to host a medical school as part of the government's expansion plans for training doctors. We cannot give you an *Insiders' Guide* to the new medical school because the first students will begin their studies in September 2003. The text following is a statement from the School.

The new Brighton and Sussex Medical School (BSMS) will accept its first intake of 128 students in Autumn 2003. BSMS is a partnership between the Universities of Brighton and Sussex and the new Brighton and Sussex University Hospitals NHS Trust. Our students will be members of both universities, and enjoy access to the academic and recreational facilities of each. The two universities have complementary strengths that will benefit the new medical school, and both have biomedical research interests recognised by grade 5 research ratings. Sussex has one of England's largest biological sciences schools, while Brighton has extensive and in-depth experience in the education and training of health professionals, including postgraduate doctors, nurses, midwives, pharmacists, physiotherapists, and medical laboratory scientists.

The two universities have adjacent campuses at Falmer, with fast rail and road links to central Brighton. Brighton, newly elevated to city status, has a vibrant social scene, to which the universities' students (over 10% of the population) make a prominent contribution. The campuses also have direct pedestrian access into the planned new South Downs National Park, long recognised as an area of outstanding natural beauty.

In your first two years your academic and clinical studies will be based in new facilities at the Falmer campuses. You will start to gain direct experience of working with patients from the first term. Clinical experience at this stage will be mainly in primary care and community medicine settings, and you will carry out two individual family studies – in year 1 with a family looking after a new baby and in year 2 with a family including a dependant requiring continuing care. You will also experience medical practice in some hospital settings, including visits to a busy A&E unit. In parallel you will develop your clinical and communication skills and study the normal and abnormal functioning of the human body using a system-based approach. The systems modules include the core material that every doctor must know, and are centred around weekly clinical symposia that employ a problem-based learning approach. They also include student-selected options that allow you to explore selected topics in greater depth, informed by the latest research.

During years 3–5 a balance between clinical and academic studies is maintained. While you gain progressively more experience in clinical contexts, the requirement to integrate your clinical experience with your understanding of the underlying clinical and social sciences and public health issues continues. You will maintain an individual clinical skills portfolio that will become an important element in the assessment of your progress, and a personal development portfolio to help you to reflect on how your personal strengths are developing along with your clinical experience. Your studies will now be based at the new Medical Education Centre at the Royal Sussex County Hospital, Brighton. Year 5 is essentially an apprenticeship year to prepare you for your postgraduate year as a Pre-Registration House Officer (PRHO). During the year you will undertake periods of regional attachment in which you will experience a rotation of clinical placements in district general hospital and community settings in Sussex and its adjoining counties. During your regional attachments you will also spend periods shadowing a PRHO.

A wide range of teaching methods are employed, with the emphasis on the small group academic and clinical teaching possible in a small and personal medical school. Individual patient studies, in which you will relate clinical findings and treatment to the principles of the underlying clinical and social sciences, will develop your understanding of the practice of medicine. We believe it is important to integrate information from different disciplines and sources, and this is emphasised throughout the curriculum.

Your degree in medicine will equip you with the knowledge, clinical skills and attitudes that you will need to progress to the next stage of your training, the PRHO year. This will normally be undertaken in hospitals and community settings within the part of the South-East region served by BSMS, and will include a formal BSMS-supervised postgraduate training programme to guide you through to full registration. Successful completion of this PRHO year will qualify you for registration with the GMC as a medical practitioner. The student-selected options within the BSMS degree will equip you to either progress to a career in general practice or to undertake postgraduate specialisation to become, after further training, a medical consultant in a clinical specialty.

Your degree will also give you real insight into the astonishing pace of development of understanding in the biomedical sciences, and prepare you for the life-long learning to which every doctor must commit themselves to keep up to date. You will gain personal experience in medical research as a member of a BSMS, Brighton or Sussex research team through your year 4 individual research project. Subject to your performance, you may also have the opportunity to extend this aspect of your study by including an intercalated BSc within your medical degree. On graduation, you will have the necessary academic background to practise evidence-based medicine and, if you wish, embark on a career combining medical practice with medical research.

In the course of your studies you will develop the key personal skills and attitudes necessary for a successful professional career, in whatever direction it may develop. These include

- Learning how to learn – especially important in a field such as medicine, where progress is so rapid that today's knowledge soon becomes obsolete
- The communication skills necessary for effective engagement with patients and fellow health professionals
- The ability to work effectively with others in multiprofessional teams to deliver first-class healthcare to individual patients and to society as a whole, and where appropriate to lead the team
- The personal and ethical attitudes essential for good professional practice and an appreciation of your responsibilities to your patients, to your professional colleagues, to society as a whole, and to yourself
- Information technology skills – you will need to learn to use a wide range of IT applications to access information and diagnostic resources and to maintain patient records.

Additional application information

Average A-level requirements	• ABB, must include chemistry or biology, both to AS-level
Average Scottish Higher requirements	• ABB at Advanced Higher, must include chemistry or biology, both to Higher level
Make-up of interview panel	• Three panel members who make independent recommendations – a member of BSMS faculty, a GP, and a third member who may be a hospital consultant, a junior doctor, or a member of another health profession
Months in which interviews are held	• November and February
Proportion of overseas students	• UK, Channel Island and EU students only
Proportion of mature students	• –
Faculty's view of students taking a gap year	• Students are welcome to apply to BSMS during year 13 for deferred entry or during the gap year itself. They must, however, be available for interview
Proportion of students taking intercalated degrees	• Provision made for intercalated year, but no students will reach this stage until 2006
Possibility of direct entrance to clinical phase	• Not at the present time
Fees for graduates	• NA
Fees for overseas students	• Does not accept overseas students yet

Further information

For further information about the Brighton and Sussex Medical School and its curriculum see its Web: http://www.bsms.ac.uk

For general information on studying at the Universities of Brighton and Sussex visit their Web: http://www.brighton.ac.uk and http://www.sussex.ac.uk, or contact the BSMS admissions office.

BSMS Admissions Undergraduate Office (Admissions)
Sussex House
University of Sussex
Falmer
Sussex BNI 9RH

University of Brighton
Mithras House
Brighton
East Sussex BN2 4AT

Tel: 01273 600900
Answerphone: 01273 642825
Fax: 01273 642828
Email: admissions@brighton.ac.uk
Web: http://www.brighton.ac.uk, http://www.sussex.ac.uk

Bristol

Key facts	Premedical	Undergraduate	Graduate course
Course length	6 years	5 years	4 years
Total number of medical students		c. 1000	
Applicants in 2002	264	1757	163
Interviews given in 2002		40%	
Places available in 2002	10	230	19
Places available in 2003	10	230	19
Entrance requirements	2:1 or AAB	AAB	2:1 BSc
Mandatory subjects	Non-science	Chemistry	Biomedical science
Male:female ratio		41:59	
Fast-track course	No	No	Yes

Bristol is one of the old red-brick universities but has a very modern and dynamic course. As well as a close-knit medical school, there are numerous opportunities to enjoy a wide circle of friends. The city centre provides an excellent and reasonably compact environment in which to work and play. The university itself has an excellent reputation, producing high-quality research and supporting good teaching. Bristol also offers a premedical year to a small number of students each year, in which the teaching is with predental students and provided by departments in the Faculty of Science. As from October 2003, Bristol will run an official (NHS bursary eligible) four-year fast-track course for graduates. There will only be 19 places and the course will only be available to Honours graduates in biosciences (see Chapter 4).

Education

Bristol introduced an integrated curriculum in 1995. The integrated course consists of three phases. Phase I, lasting two terms, acts as an introductory period and provides a basic understanding of the human body and the mechanisms of health and disease (molecular and cellular basis of medicine). Phase I also has a human basis of medicine component, where students learn medical sociology, ethics, and epidemiology. This is mainly taught in the School of Medical Sciences. Phase II lasts until the end of the third year and consists of mixed clinical and theory-based systems-orientated teaching. Phase III includes teaching and clinical experience of specialty subjects (such as paediatrics, obstetrics, and gynaecology). In addition, phase III includes the elective period and senior clinical attachments in medicine and surgery. Clinical contact begins in general practices in the first year, and the first hospital attachment is in the second year. During phases II and III the whole year group is regularly brought together in Bristol for lectures and tutorial teaching.

Teaching

Early-phase teaching consists mainly of lectures and practicals, supplemented by small group tutorials and some self-directed learning. (No live animals are used in practicals, though occasionally some tissue, such as crab legs and guinea-pig ileum, is used in experiments.) Topographical anatomy is taught by young medical demonstrators using cadaveric prosections. Students have the opportunity to do a short dissection project in anatomy in their second year. Anatomy is a popular and rewarding element of the medical degree course at Bristol.

Assessment

Regular assessments are made throughout the course. Many clinical attachments include projects or the preparation and delivery of a case presentation, whereas science teaching carries associated tutorial and practical work. There are usually exams at the end of each year, although continuous assessment contributes to the final-year mark. There are important exams at the end of the third year, and finals at the end of the fifth year.

Intercalated degrees

Undertaking a BSc is a popular option, with about 30% of students opting to intercalate. The school positively encourages students to intercalate, usually after the second year, but it is possible to do so after the third year. Students may choose a conventional science subject, such as biochemistry or pathology, although recently programmes such as bioethics have been introduced. The Honours year gives students an opportunity to try some "real" science in the form of a potentially publishable original research project, as opposed to the rather structured medical course.

Special study modules and electives

SSMs are an important part of the new curriculum from the first year onwards, allowing students to pursue subjects of special interest. Elective time is currently eight weeks at the beginning of the fifth year.

Facilities

Library The medical library is open until 9 pm on weekdays (5 pm or 6 pm during the long vacation) and on Saturdays. The main library has longer opening hours. Popular textbooks are available from the medical library on a short loan basis. Medline, Embase and other databases are on open access on library computers, and email and internet connection are also available there and in the halls of residence.

Computers   Computers are available in the medical school (including the library) and in the main library. There are a number of 24-hour open-access rooms dotted around the university. Computer-assisted learning packages are available in the medical library. Other terminals support internet access, email, word processing, etc. Information technology is supposed to be an integral part of the new course, but the quality of computing facilities is variable.

Clinical skills   All the teaching centres have facilities, though the primary site is in one of the main teaching hospitals in Bristol, the Bristol Royal Infirmary. In the second year adult life support is taught and students are examined and certified. The clinical skills laboratory is also used to teach venepuncture to second-year students. As students progress through the course, other clinical procedures, such as intubation, may be learnt here or in the medical academies (see 'placements').

Welfare

Student support

There is a personal tutor scheme in operation and it normally works well, the quality of the scheme depending on both the tutor (and the tutee). However, most students find a member of staff with whom they get on well and from whom they can seek help. The faculty tends to be supportive, provided they are informed of problems before they get out of hand. There is a staff–student liaison committee, but input does not often translate into immediate action. The university and the Students' Union both have counselling services. Access for students with disabilities may be difficult because of the layout of the university (on a steep hill). The secretary of Galenicals (the medical students' society) is also there to voice student opinions and views to the medical school.

Accommodation

Most first-years are accommodated in university halls of residence. These tend to be comfortable enough and provide an excellent opportunity to bond with other freshers (medics and non-medics) at the numerous organised events or in the hall bars. The main group of halls is located a 30–40-minute walk from the university precinct. It is possible to apply to stay in hall after the first year, but most people move into university flats/houses or into accommodation in the private sector. Weekly rents vary between £50 and £60 or more, but most students pay between £55 and £60. It is usual to pay rent over the summer and the scrum for houses starts quite early in the year. The accommodation office provides some help, but a lot depends on individual initiative.

Placements

The first two years are spent mainly around the university campus in central Bristol. When you begin clinical specialty attachments you can be placed at one of the main Bristol hospitals or anywhere within a 50-mile radius of Bristol. Attachments are from the third year onward and will usually be within 50 miles of Bristol. Medical academies are being established in Taunton, Bath, Cheltenham, Swindon, and Gloucester. The concept of an academy is a group of teachers and students (up to 80) focused on medical school activities and with equivalent resources to the home university. Students will usually spend six months at each academy, and during the three years half the time will be located in academies within Bristol. General practice attachments are also spread across the southwest. Accommodation is provided wherever it is essential for students to be away from Bristol. However, although some help is given with travel expenses, travel to and from these attachments can be an extra expense (especially if you want to come back every weekend).

Sports and social

City life

Bristol has a lot to offer both as a university and as a city. The university is a research-orientated institution with a good reputation but also provides good teaching. The city is just brilliant fun. Mainstream attractions abound and there is plenty of "alternative" entertainment for those who want it. It is still reasonably safe (at least in the areas frequented by students), provided appropriate precautions are taken. It is certainly no worse than most other cities in this respect. If city life becomes too hectic, there are plenty of green spaces to escape to.

The city centre is reasonably compact and packed with things to attract all comers. The countryside (and the attractions of the West Country and Wales) is not far away. Students tend to congregate in the areas just around the university, such as Clifton. However, there is a shift towards areas a little further away which offer cheaper rents. Clifton is the most affluent (and "posey") part of Bristol, offering pleasant cafes and bijou shops. "Town and gown" tension is rarely a problem. Shopping, theatre, museum and music lovers will all find something up their street. There are plenty of pubs, restaurants, clubs, cinemas (including three "arthouse" cinemas), plenty of parks and green spaces, and all the other things you would associate with a vibrant city like Bristol.

Uni life

Entertainment abounds in Bristol – sometimes there seems to be too much choice! A number of big acts play at the university and at other venues throughout the city. There is a huge range of societies to join at the Union. Halls and Galenicals lay on a range of entertainment, organise a number of sports teams, and represent students' views on a variety of committees. There are two revues for medics to take part in. The preclinical revue tends to be a rather drunken and disorganised affair, but the clinical one is a more organised and moderate event that runs for four nights in the Union theatre. Galenicals organises a lot of events for medics and has its own bar which students from all year groups use.

Sports life

The university has good outdoor facilities, a new indoor tennis centre, and plans are well under way to develop a new indoor centre within the campus. Wednesday afternoons are usually free for sport, and there are teams at all levels in most sports. There are a number of medics' teams (including the infamous Women's Football Team) organised through Galenicals, which tend to be a bit less competitive than the university teams. They have a considerable social component (and alcohol consumption, too!).

Great things about Bristol

- Friendly and close-knit.
- The generally high standard of teaching and the high quality of clinical experience, especially in peripheral hospitals.
- The city of Bristol itself, with its huge range of bars, restaurants and attractions.
- The opportunity to mix with plenty of non-medics and medics from other year groups.
- A modern, clinical course in which student feedback is valued.

Bad things about Bristol

- The rather conservative nature of the university in terms of atmosphere and politics.
- The financial costs (high rents; long distance attachments in clinical years; expensive bus fares).
- Walking up all those steep hills (Bristol is one big hill).
- Feedback on exams you have just taken can sometimes be a bit limited.
- Huge annual scramble for accommodation at a reasonable price.

Additional application information	
Average A-level requirements	• AAB, including chemistry
Average Scottish Higher requirements	• Please check with admissions office
Make-up of interview panel	• Academics/NHS clinicians
Months in which interviews are held	• November–March
Proportion of overseas students	• 5%
Proportion of mature students	• 15%
Faculty's view of students taking a gap year	• Positive if used well
Proportion of students taking intercalated degrees	• 30%
Possibility of direct entrance to clinical phase	• No
Fees for graduates	• £1100
Fees for overseas students	• £10 105 pa (preclinical) and £18 715 pa (clinical)
Assistance for elective funding	• No
Assistance for travel to attachments	• Some
Access and hardship funds	• Some grants and bursaries
Weekly rent	• Halls £34–£90 Private £45-£70
Pint of lager	• Union bar £1.50 City centre pub £2.20
Cinema	• £3–£5
Nightclub	• Free–£8

Further information

Undergraduate Admissions Office
University of Bristol
Senate House
Tyndall Avenue
Bristol BS8 ITH
Tel: 0117 928 7679
Fax: 0117 925 1424
Email: admissions@bristol.ac.uk
Web: http://www.medici.bris.ac.uk

Cambridge

Key facts	Undergraduate course	Graduate entry
Course length	5½ years	4 years
Total number of medical students	c. 1200	40
Applicants in 2002	1189	
Interviews given in 2002	96%	
Places available in 2002	268	20
Places available in 2003	268	20
Entrance requirements	AAA	2:1 degree
Mandatory subjects	Chemistry and biology	Med & Vet Admissions Test
Male:female ratio	47:53	
Premed course	No	No
Fast-track course	No	Yes

The Cambridge undergraduate course follows the traditional format for medical education, which places much emphasis on understanding the principles behind biological science and its application to medical practice and research. What makes the Cambridge course very different from most others is the supervision system at both the preclinical and the clinical stages. The medics tend to be a very social group, mixing work and play quite effectively. The course is quite intense; however, there is ample opportunity for extracurricular activities, not just within the colleges but also in the university and within the city itself.

Education

The course is clearly separated into the preclinical and clinical stages. The preclinical course (Phase I) is divided into two parts. Parts Ia and Ib (years 1 and 2) concentrate on basic medical sciences such as anatomy, histology, and pharmacology, in addition to preparing students to deal with patients. It is essential to gain second MB exemptions (at least a 2:2) in these subjects in order to enter the clinical phase in the fourth year.

Phase II (third year) is the compulsory BA (Hons). Project options in the third year are usually medically related. However, one of the advantages of the Cambridge course is that it is possible to take a break from medicine and study a completely different discipline, such as law, theology, management studies, and even physics (if daring). In addition, there are two further "preparing for patients" strands during this year.

The clinical stage, which is based at Addenbrooke's Hospital, is intensive, lasting only 27 months, and is divided into three phases, during which time attachments to all the major specialties are organised. Final MB examinations in pathology and obstetrics and gynaecology are taken at the end of Phase II (after 18 months of the clinical course) and the remainder at the end of Phase III. Most of the work is ward based and students are expected to be proactive. There are lecture blocks throughout the course, but these are kept to a minimum. It should be remembered that there is non-automatic progression to the clinical school and only about half the Cambridge preclinical students stay on, although last year all students who wanted to stay on were able to do so. The rest normally go to the London schools or Oxford, but it is also possible to go to Edinburgh or other medical schools with compatible courses to undertake clinical studies.

The university now sets a two-hour admission test for all applicants to all colleges. This is taken at the student's own school. It consists of multiple choice questions (sections A and B) and two essays from maths, biology, chemistry or physics subject areas. The test is designed to make you think and reason clearly about particular topics and is not a test of factual knowledge. It requires no knowledge beyond key stage 4 of the National Curriculum, and should not stop anyone from coming here. Everyone who applies is still interviewed, and for the next couple of years the examiners do not intend the test result to form a large part of the criteria upon which the offer of a place is made.

Teaching

During the preclinical stage the teaching programme consists of lectures (with the occasional seminar) and practicals (which must be attended) organised by the medical sciences departments. These are supplemented by weekly small group tutorials (consisting of two or three students) known as supervisions, which are organised by the individual colleges. The majority of teaching in the clinical stage is ward based. Some emphasis is placed on computer-assisted methods of learning, and students are expected to be reasonably computer literate by the end of the course.

Assessment

This takes the form of end-of-year examinations. These are essay or theoretical experimental practical papers, but a few are actually practical papers. During the functional architecture of the body course there are occasional informal "sign-up" or viva tests which do not contribute to the end-of-year grade but ensure that you are keeping up to date with the work. In Phase II, a research project or dissertation may contribute to your classification. Assessment of progress in the clinical years is at the end of most attachments. Formal assessment, vivas, and written exams take place at the end of each phase. A doctor arranges weekly clinical supervisions to monitor/guide the student through the entire course.

Intercalated degrees

All students must complete the third year (Phase II), which leads to a BA (Hons) in the subject in which they have specialised.

Special study modules and electives

The elective study takes place after the final MB exams at the end of Phase II. It is seven weeks in duration and 95% of students go abroad. Limited funding is available for electives from the clinical school and possibly from your college, although students have to compete for these (value £80–£200, total £2000), and there may also be some assistance from your college (value dependent on the college).

Facilities

Library Not finding a library in Cambridge would be like not finding a single Italian restaurant in Rome. All libraries are fairly central, and all colleges, departments and faculties will have their own collections as well. There is also a central university library, a central city library, and a specialist medical library at the clinical school, therefore the last excuse one can use is that you could not find it in any of the libraries! All of the libraries are open during office hours, and some have 24-hour access.

Computers As with the libraries, there are computing facilities everywhere; everyone is given an email account (cam.ac.uk) as well as college and university logins. Most colleges have university network connections to some of the undergraduate rooms. Computer services for students at Cambridge are excellent.

Welfare

Student support

Administration of the preclinical course is at college and university level, but all students are given a tutor (a non-medical Fellow), who is responsible for their pastoral care, and a director of studies (medical Fellow) who is concerned with ensuring they receive the appropriate academic help. The Clinical Dean is also friendly and helpful.

Accommodation

Quality and cost vary with the college (and the wealth of the college), so choose wisely, especially if you are a clinical or overseas student. All of the colleges will provide accommodation in or close to college for the preclinical years, and most will provide accommodation for the clinical years. The standard at its worst is definitely bearable. At its best you are unlikely to get better rooms anywhere else, and it is probably better than your own room at home! Additionally, the majority of colleges have "bedders" who clean rooms – it would obviously be a waste of valuable study time to do your own cleaning. During the clinical stage you may have to rent accommodation from local landlords and this costs between £50 and £60 per week for a middle-of-the-range house, usually shared by three or four people.

Placements

The preclinical lectures, seminars and practicals are all held in the Science Faculty away from the hospital, and all within walking distance of the central colleges. The tutorials are usually held within your own college. Very few teaching sessions are held in the hospital during the preclinical stage. During the clinical stage all the teaching is done at Addenbrooke's, which is situated 2½ miles from the city centre and can be easily reached by bus or bicycle (30 minutes) if you are not able to force a friend to give you a lift.

There are regional attachments in up to a maximum of six out of the 11 Phase I and II placements. In Phase III, half of the time is spent at Addenbrooke's and half in a district general hospital. Accommodation at these placements is provided. Students are usually allocated attachments; however, if a student is heavily involved in a university sport they can arrange to remain in Addenbrooke's for the majority of firms.

Sports and social

City life

With its undeniable beauty and rich history, Cambridge is an inspiring city to work and live in. Undergraduates during term time, graduates and tourists at all times and, of course, the local residents (affectionately known as "townies") provide an ever-changing and colourful population superimposed on secluded college cloisters, colonies of student houses, and a busy town centre. On a more practical note, all the usual student needs are provided for within a 15-minute cycle ride or less. Take your pick from the covered central market, essential supermarkets, and a wide range of chain stores, the excellent Arts Theatre, Corn Exchange and Guildhall, as well as a number of cinemas – college, arthouse and mainstream. The river soon meanders to open countryside in either direction and, finally, many routes lead out of Cambridge to London (and its attractions) as well as the rest of the country.

Cambridge is not without the dangers of violence and crime and, like most places, these problems are often associated with last orders on a Friday or Saturday night. However, there are no notorious districts and students' property insurance premiums confirm Cambridge as one of the safest places to live and study.

Uni life

Cambridge life is a heady mix in terms of inhabitants and surroundings. The collegiate system means that in the preclinical years you get to meet students doing a wide variety of subjects, and not just medics. Although the course does place a workload on you there is time to do plenty of other things, such as sport – in particular rowing – and music, which are well represented throughout the university. There is much more of a "medical school" feel to the clinical stage, with most students living nearer the hospital and away from their colleges. The small year group sizes mean that by the end of the course everyone gets to know one another.

Entertainments are provided at a variety of levels, and may be society, college, clinical school or university based. If that is not enough, then there are many shows and concerts put on by non-university establishments in the town. Cambridge is very different from other universities in that there is no central Student Union bar where everyone accumulates. There are bars in each college and student nights during the week at the various Cambridge hot spots. Formal halls are a prominent feature of the Cambridge social scene. This is a three-course meal costing between £3 and £5. Students wear gowns, Latin is muttered and a gong sounds. It is hard to believe this becomes normality, but it's great fun and brilliant to keep tradition alive; it's just a nightmare when it's five minutes before graduation and you find three-year-old food ingrained in your gown!

The University Medical Society is the fourth largest and works to make sure medics have a good time. Every year there is a Christmas dinner, and other activities such as bops, barbecues and pub crawls are also organised. In addition, each college has its own medical society which hosts a number of dinners each year and provides ample opportunity to socialise on a less academic level with fellows. Finally, sporting (drinking) societies play a large part in Cambridge social life. This often involves a bizarre initiation, for example eating dog food off crackers, and you are then entitled to name yourself a Wench, Strumpet, Roo, etc., depending on the college/society. Drinking societies collaborate and one society will host a formal hall in their college and invite a drinking society of the opposite sex to join them. It's an excellent way of networking and meeting individuals from different colleges studying different subjects. It also serves as a large-scale dating agency! On top of this, there is a whole host of opportunities to be involved in other societies, from drama (the famous Cambridge Footlights) and music to karate and gliding, so the chances are you can find something you will enjoy doing.

Sports life

Almost every sport is catered for at the university level. Facilities at college level vary, but at best include huge playing fields, a multigym, and squash courts. Boat clubs, football, rugby, and cricket tend to have the largest shares of the college budgets. Also, it does not matter how good or bad you are, there is always an opportunity to take part in whatever you choose. During the preclinical stage sport is college based and there is fierce intercollegiate rivalry. The clinical school has a sports society (known as "the Sharks") and there is a sport and fitness centre situated on the hospital site to which all students are given free membership.

Finally, another popular sport in Cambridge is punting. Whether you like to get physical or simply recline, enjoying the cool breeze and listening to punt chauffeurs telling elaborate lies to awestruck tourists, you will love punting!

Great things about Cambridge

- The collegiate system means that you get to meet students doing a wide variety of subjects.
- The supervision and tutorial system ensures that you are able to get help with any academic difficulties, helps to make sure that you are able to keep up with the course, and gives you substantially more individual tuition than most medical schools. It also makes sure you do the work!
- The social life in Cambridge is brilliant. Every society and college hosts dinners and events, and there is always something to do.

- May week! Actually in June, after the preclinical exams. A week of celebrating, winding down, and college balls! After all this, you have three months (in the preclinical years) to skip off into the sunset completely free of work worries.
- The cost of living is relatively low, and the proximity of all the necessary amenities makes Cambridge an ideal place to spend life as a student. Additionally, there are many funds/bursaries available to all students for travel, study and extracurricular activities. In light of the proposed financial adjustments for students attending university, Cambridge will be attractive to anyone who might struggle financially.

Bad things about Cambridge

- Cambridge is highly academic and can appear to be a very competitive learning environment, especially just prior to exams, which for some students can be rather stressful. It is common to have five hours to complete three essays, a rowing outing in 10 minutes, and a thumping head from the previous night's antics. This is known as "fifth week blues" and affects most students.
- Living in halls for the first three years can be frustrating, as the rules and regulations the college enforces can make some individuals feel as though they are not being treated like an adult. However, this is a trade-off for having cheap accommodation without the hassle of deposits, landlords, and paying utility bills.
- The course is intensive and it may be easy to fall behind. Although the preclinical terms are short (only eight weeks of study) they can be very tiring, but this is made up for by longer holidays.
- The small size of the town can make life feel somewhat claustrophobic at times, especially after three years of study.
- The tourists – though admittedly they do generate a lot of income for the town and the colleges – tend to get under your skin and manage to appear almost anywhere and at any time (including occasionally in lectures!).

Additional application information	
Average A-level requirements	• AAA in sciences/maths – some colleges ask for STEP papers
Average Scottish Higher requirements	• Check with individual college admissions tutors
Make-up of interview panel	• This varies from college to college, from being very informal to having written tests; 2–4 interviews may be required
Months in which interviews are held	• December, prior to A-levels
Proportion of overseas students	• 18 per year
Proportion of mature students	• 12 per year
Faculty's view of students taking a gap year	• Dependent on individual college
Proportion of students taking intercalated degrees	• None; all students study for three preclinical years, including BA (Hons)
Possibility of direct entrance to clinical phase	• All students are interviewed again before entry to clinical school. About 10% of the clinical school's intake is from other UK medical schools
Fees for graduates	• £2805 pa
Fees for overseas students	• Preclinical approx £9500 pa Clinical £17 500 pa plus £3000 for non-domiciled
Assistance for elective funding	• There are a limited number of bursaries
Assistance for travel to attachments	• Only available to LEA-funded students
Access and hardship funds	• Dependent on individual college
Weekly rent	• Halls £40–£60 Private £40–£75
Pint of lager	• Union/college bar £1.50 City centre pub: £2.10
Cinema	• £1.50–£3.80 (with student card)
Nightclub	• Free–£15

Further information

University of Cambridge
The Clinical School
Addenbrooke's Hospital
Hills Road
Cambridge CB2 2SP
Tel: 01223 336700
Email: ucam-undergraduate-admissions@lists.ca.ac.uk
Web: http://www.medschl.cam.ac.uk

Dundee

Key facts	Dundee
Course length	5 years
Total number of medical undergraduates	c. 800
Applicants in 2002	1337
Interviews given in 2002	37%
Places available in 2002	154
Places available in 2003	154
Entrance requirements	ABB
Mandatory subjects	Chemistry
Male:female ratio	45:55
Premed course	Yes
Fast-track course	No

Dundee is a progressive, modern, friendly, forward-thinking medical school with an international reputation. The new curriculum was introduced in 1993. Dundee medics have a reputation for being friendly and down to earth. Intake is approximately 40% Scottish, 40% Irish, 10% English, and 10% overseas. Dundee is extremely supportive of graduate/mature students and encourages applications from a wide variety of backgrounds. Over 16% of every year are graduate/mature students, and each year also has about seven entrants from the premed course. The curriculum offers good staff–student participation and has achievable learning goals with a realistic workload. Clinical teaching begins in the second year. Many aspects of the course at Dundee have received plaudits from the Scottish Higher Education Funding Council. The biomedical research programme is world renowned. Ninewells Hospital, the largest purpose-built teaching hospital in Europe, is built on a green park campus on the banks of the River Tay.

Education

The first cohort from the new-style course graduated in 2000 and the integrated course is well established. Teaching is structured around body systems. The first year (Phase I) covers normal body structure and function and is taught at the main campus. First-year students also visit patients in the community and do a basic CPR (cardiopulmonary resuscitation) course. During the first year students are divided into groups for tutorials and practicals. Groups change in the second year for the Practising Medicine (clinical) programme, which helps you get to know more of your year. Phase II (second and third years) and III (fourth and fifth years) are based at Ninewells Hospital. The curriculum requires mastery (a pass grade of 75%) of relevant facts, clinical skills, and attitude. Special study modules are a key component, but are assessed using different criteria.

Teaching

The systems-based course promotes independent learning. Each block comes with a study guide, which includes core material and a summary of the clinical skills to be mastered each week, problem-based questions, tutorial questions and references. Phase I teaching is a mixture of lectures, dissection, laboratories, behavioural sciences, and tutorials. There is no use of animals or animal tissues in practicals. Phase II includes clinical skills, ward teaching (about eight students to a ward group), small group work, and primary care medicine.

Phase III is primarily clinical and includes a house officer apprenticeship in the fifth year. This provides extensive training so that students will be competent and useful house officers, and often occurs in the hospital where the PRHO year will be spent. Multidisciplinary teaching takes place between the medical and nursing schools for ethics, and between the medical and midwifery schools for some parts of the Phase II reproduction, growth, and development block. Teaching at Dundee has recently been rated excellent by the Scottish Higher Education Funding Council and is well thought of in GMC assessments.

Assessment

Traditional finals have been replaced with short exams and portfolio assessment. Phase exams are made up of extended matching questions and problem-based type questions and an objective structured clinical exam (OSCE).

Intercalated degrees

Students take an intercalated degree by invitation from faculty. Subjects typically include medical/social sciences, but BAs can also be taken. Dundee is the only school to offer a BMSc in forensic medicine and orthopaedic technology. A few students take a degree at one of the London schools.

Special study modules and electives

Over 42 SSMs are advertised on the medical school website, or you can design your own – overseas options are available. Staff are very supportive of individually designed SSMs happening in their clinics/laboratories. Fifth year kicks off with a seven-week elective (10 weeks if you tack on your three-week vacation!). It's up to you to organise your own programme. Information and help regarding funding are widely available.

Facilities

Library   Year 1 books are housed in a large multifaculty library on the main campus. Years 2–5 books are housed at Ninewells Hospital Library. Normal opening hours are Monday to Friday 9 am–10 pm; Saturday and Sunday 9 am–6 pm. There is good availability of reference books, but be prepared to reserve some books in advance. Libraries open later as the academic year progresses.

Computers   There is extensive computer access at both Ninewells (open 8 am–11 pm all week) and the main campus. Facilities include computer-assisted learning (CAL) tutorials, microbiology laboratory summaries, MCQs, MRI/CT/X-ray imaging, revision sessions, email and internet. Classes in IT skills are laid on for the nervous!

Clinical skills   The purpose-built clinical skills centre opened in 1997. It provides multiprofessional and multidisciplinary teaching to small groups in areas such as communication and history taking; professional attitudes and ethics; physical examination and laboratory skills; diagnostics and therapeutics; and resuscitation. The centre is open 9 am–5 pm for teaching and drop-in revision sessions. The clinical and administrative staff are extremely supportive and proactive, and run a book-in service for revising clinical skills. Facilities include access to anatomical models and mannequins; diagnostic, therapeutic and resuscitation equipment; videos; simulated and real patients; and telemedicine links. Typical clinical skills sessions in Phase II (years 2 and 3) are generally good fun, last two hours, and allow students to develop confidence and competence in clinical skills before going on to the wards.

Welfare

Student support

The staff tend to be friendly, approachable, and supportive. They really do make an effort to ensure that students get the extra clinical training, core knowledge, and time for small group work required by the new curriculum. A new staff–student leisure facility at Ninewells was completed in 1998, and a house officer facility was completed in 1996. The School of Nursing and Midwifery joined the Faculty of Medicine and Dentistry in 1997. Each student is assigned a personal and academic tutor. There is a Special Needs Coordinator, based at Student Welfare on the main campus. The Dean is very approachable and student friendly, and operates an open-door policy. Likewise, lecturers and clinicians are approachable, and typically put a lot of work into designing and teaching each systems block. All medical freshers are sent a student-produced *Student Survival Guide*, which covers academics, social, sport, local transport, etc. The students run a Senior–Junior scheme. There is also a very active Medical Students' Council, which regularly attends faculty meetings to voice student opinion. The council also runs a careers fair, women in medicine, annual symposium, electives, and PRHO meetings for students. A good indicator of staff–student relations is the number of staff who regularly attend year club and hospital balls. The medical school has good wheelchair access.

Accommodation

There are two halls on campus. Belmont is a large 1900s catered hall of residence next to the Union, the sports centre, and the library. Airlie is a smaller self-catering hall on the other side of the Union and the library. Peterson House and Seabraes Flats are a one-minute stumble from campus. They are both self-catering; the latter was built in 1996, with flats with en-suite bathrooms, etc. The West Park Centre is halfway between the town and Ninewells in the leafy west end of Dundee, and offers both catered and self-catering halls. This accommodation was also built in 1996, and has self-contained flats with phones, en-suite bathrooms, colour TVs and computer links to the university internet. Most first-years live in hall. Private accommodation costs about £40–50 per week, generally in the west end of Dundee, and standards are pretty good.

Placements

The first year is based at the main campus, in the city centre. Years 2–5 are hospital based. Ninewells Hospital is about three miles from the town and main campus on the Firth of Tay. Wards have spectacular river views. Many students walk (30 minutes), cycle, or drive in but numerous buses run right to the front door (fare 95p). Car parking is available but is expensive.

In the second and third years ward teaching is at Ninewells Hospital. Some teaching is at Perth Royal Infirmary, 20 miles away. In the fourth and fifth years you get a chance to travel around the UK and see how other hospitals work: up to five months of the fourth and fifth years can be spent away from Dundee on outblocks if desired. Placements with district general hospitals (DGHs) and GPs are set up around Scotland (including the Highlands and Islands) and the north of England, with free hospital accommodation provided. Guesthouse accommodation or travel expenses are available for many GP placements. A computer matching system allocates students to their peripheral attachments, so most students can stay in Dundee if they wish, although for many the experience of peripheral hospital/GP attachments is a highlight.

Sports and social

City life

Dundee is Scotland's fourth largest city and has a beautiful location on the Firth of Tay. Local sights include the riverside itself; the neighbouring seaside town of Broughty Ferry with its sandy beaches, castle, shops and pubs; Tentsmuir Forest Park and beaches; Carnoustie; St Andrews (15 miles away); numerous golf courses; and fantastic sunsets. As well as being spectacular, the countryside offers skiing, hill walking, climbing, and numerous water sports. A new shopping centre opened in 2000, vastly improving Dundee's shopping facilities. The city is very student friendly, and the area around the university is very much a student community. Many new small shops, cafés, bars, and clubs have opened over the past 18 months. There is constant building and renovation work in the town. Glasgow, Edinburgh, and Aberdeen are all within reach for a weekend, from a 1–1½-hour drive/train journey away.

Uni life

Dundee University Medical Society (DUMS) sponsors freshers' week events, and puts on many social bashes and trips throughout the year. DUMS tends to form a large part of a medic's social life, especially in the earlier years. Each year also has its own year club to put on events – for example end of year balls, fancy dress parties, nights out, pub golf and slave auctions – to raise money for charity. Ceilidhs (Scottish dancing) are very popular and are a great ice-breaker. Lessons are given for the uninitiated. Each year club organises a halfway dinner (weekend away with ball, etc.) guess when – halfway through the course – and their own graduation ball (there is also a university graduation ball). The Students Union building has been refurbished and hosts packed-out club nights through the week, and is very popular with medics. Local pubs abound (some hosting live music) and the beer is cheap. The Dundee Repertory Theatre is active nationally, and hosts plays, musicals, and jazz festivals. The popular Dundee Contemporary Arts Centre provides two screens for "arthouse" films, a large art gallery, café and wine bar, all right beside the university. There are two multiplex cinemas and an arthouse cinema. The Duncan of Jordanstone Art School is part of the main campus, adding diversity to the student population, and their summer final-year show is always a sell-out. The university also has the usual wide variety of societies and sporting organisations.

Sports life

The sports centre now boasts the largest university indoor facilities in Scotland. Outdoor pitches are based at the scenic and windy Riverside Drive. The university has a very active and varied sports scene, with a good level of competition in both Scottish and British university systems. The medical school has its own mixed teams in hockey, basketball, and volleyball, with single-sex teams in football, rugby, and netball. Competitions are organised against other Scottish medical schools. Medics often play for both the medical school and the university, with the medical school teams being a little less competitive in spirit than the university teams. A number of non-competitive trips and activities are open to all students and staff, such as sailing, hill walking, climbing, ceilidh lessons, skiing, and outdoor pursuit weekends. Everybody is welcome, from beginners to the experienced.

Great things about Dundee

- Good teaching on an established new-style course.
- Good social life based around the MedSoc (DUMS) and a friendly bunch of staff and students means that you can always find something to do.
- Dundee is a cheap, safe, and nice place to live.
- The clinical skills centre is excellent.
- Dundee is surrounded by beautiful countryside, with access to skiing, hill walking, and watersports.

Bad things about Dundee

- It can take some time to get used to the local accent.
- During the fourth and fifth years the attachments mean that the year group does not meet up very often.
- Dundee is not a great centre for shopping.

- From year 2 onwards you are based almost exclusively at Ninewells and may feel a little isolated from ordinary students and student life.
- It does get cold and windy.

Additional application information

Average A-level requirements	• ABB (chemistry)
Average Scottish Higher requirements	• AAABB (chemistry)
Make-up of interview panel	• Members of the Faculty of Medicine
Months in which interviews are held	• December-March
Proportion of overseas students	• 8%
Proportion of mature students	• 10% (includes graduate entrants)
Faculty's view of students taking a gap year	• Acceptable
Proportion of students taking intercalated degrees	• 10%
Possibility of direct entrance to clinical phase	• None
Fees for graduates	• See Chapter 6
Fees for overseas students	• £11 800 pa (preclinical) and £18 800 pa (clinical)
Assistance for elective funding	• Yes – competitively every year some 20 awards are made £200 min – £1000 max
Assistance for travel to attachments	• No – responsibility of LEA
Access and hardship funds	• Yes – grants and loans available with medical school
Weekly rent	• Halls £68 Private £40–£50
Pint of lager	• Union bar £1.20 City centre pub £1.50 +
Cinema	• £3 student night, £4 other; two multiplex with 10 screens each and one arthouse cinema
Nightclub	• £2.50 Large selection offering all tastes in music/dance and entertainment

Further information

Information Centre
Admissions and Student Recruitment
2 Airlie Place
The University of Dundee
Nethergate
Dundee DD1 4HN
Tel: 01382 344160
Fax: 01382 348150
Email: srs@dundee.ac.uk
Web: http://www.dundee.ac.uk

East Anglia

Key facts	East Anglia
Course length	5 years
Total number of medical undergraduates	
Applicants in 2002	
Interviews given in 2002	
Places available in 2002	110
Places available in 2003	110
Entrance requirements	AAB
Mandatory subjects	Biology
Male:female ratio	–
Premed course	No
Fast-track course	No

The University of East Anglia (UEA) in Norwich will play host to one of the new medical schools. We cannot give you an *Insiders' Guide* to UEA Medical School because the first students only started their studies there in September 2002. The following is a statement from the school.

A brand new medical school is being launched at UEA and will offer an innovative five-year degree programme starting in September 2002. We are committed to equipping our students with an appropriate range of skills and knowledge for medical practice in the 21st century, and our curriculum reflects the latest developments in medical education. Initially there will be 110 places.

Successful applications will usually need to have three A-levels (typical offer AAB), or their equivalent if offering other qualifications. In particular, we expect candidates to demonstrate a sound knowledge of biological sciences (grade A at A-level, or equivalent), as well as academic attainment and potential in a range of scientific or other subjects. Normally at least five subjects, including both English and mathematics, should have been passed at grade A or B at GCSE or its equivalent. We welcome applications from graduates in any subject (although proof of a sound knowledge of the biological sciences will be required) and from other mature candidates with qualifications differing from those of school leavers. Entry from approved Access courses will be particularly encouraged. If you are not a home/EU student, please contact our Admissions Office before applying.

No offer will be made without an interview, during which reasons for wishing to study medicine will be explored. Satisfactory medical and police screening will be required.

As a new medical school we are working closely with the General Medical Council, which is responsible for validating our programme. Some details may change as our plans develop, but core principles are as follows.

In our curriculum, relevant skills and knowledge – including clinical and life sciences, as well as socioeconomic aspects (for example, sociology, psychology, epidemiology, management, health economics, law, and ethics) – will be studied in relation to particular clinical conditions and the ways in which patients display them to doctors. These clinical presentations are grouped into units of learning based upon body systems (for example, circulation).

To ensure a proper integration between theory and practice, students will spend a substantial part of each year gaining clinical experience with patients, in both secondary care (for example, hospitals) and primary care (that is, with GPs in health centres throughout the area). Where appropriate, experience of tertiary care (that is, specialist centres) will also be provided. The nature and extent of this integration is one the most distinctive features of our course.

As well as covering the core medical curriculum, students will have the opportunity throughout to study areas of special interest in more depth and, in later years, to take some courses in subjects outside medicine. In the fourth year there is an elective clinical placement period of eight weeks in which each student chooses the type and location of clinical experience.

Our programme offers a variety of formats and experiences to encourage student learning. Whole-class discussions, lectures, seminars – and, especially, small-group sessions – are featured in our timetable. Clinical, communication, and IT skills are taught throughout the course. Ample time is permitted for independent study. At the end of each of the first four years there is an integrative period to enable consolidation of the course to date. A similar period at the end of the final year is specifically set aside as preparation for employment as preregistration house officers after graduation.

Assessment is on a unit-by-unit basis: there are no final examinations. Arrangements include multiple-choice questionnaires; portfolios, presentations, and projects; "advanced notice" questions in which research answers need to be presented under examination conditions; and objective structured clinical examinations (OSCEs).

Academic years (excluding breaks) are provisionally 32 weeks for year 1, 39 weeks for each of years 2–4, and 33 weeks for year 5.

After graduation

As far as is practicable, UEA graduates will be employed as PRHOs by our NHS partners (in hospitals and in general practice), so that we can offer mentoring and postgraduate study during the year.

Facilities

A new, specially designed building is being constructed for the medical school at UEA. In addition, the school will make extensive use of the leading-edge facilities at the new Norfolk and Norwich Hospital – which is very close to the university campus – as well as other hospitals, GP premises, and healthcare facilities across the region.

Residential accommodation on UEA's attractive campus is guaranteed to first-year students (en-suite options available). There is good private-sector provision of houses, flats and bedsits in Norwich, a city which – while big enough to offer all the facilities of a major commercial and cultural centre – still manages to be a friendly, easy-going and safe place to live.

Further information

The Admissions Office
School of Medicine
University of East Anglia
Norwich
Norfolk
Tel: 01603 591072
Fax: 01603 593752
Email: med.admiss@uea.ac.uk
Web: http://www.uea.ac.uk

Open days: June

Edinburgh

Key facts	Edinburgh
Course length	5 years
Total number of medical undergraduates	c. 1350
Applicants in 2002	2167
Interviews given in 2002	<5% (mainly graduates, mature and widening access applicants)
Places available in 2002	218 (202 home, 16 overseas)
Places available in 2003	218
Entrance requirements	AAAB (3 A-levels, 1 AS) or AAAAB (Highers)
Mandatory subjects	Chemistry
Male:female ratio	35:65
Premed course	Yes
Fast-track course	No

Although it is one of the oldest medical schools, Edinburgh has shed the traditional preclinical/clinical course for a new integrated curriculum that started in October 1998. With a strong research tradition (reflected by 40% of students taking an intercalated BSc), Edinburgh seems to attract high academic achievers and a lot of students from England and Northern Ireland. The medical school is situated centrally, which means that you mix well with other students and feel a real part of the university and the city itself – a compact yet varied centre to escape into.

Education

The new curriculum is taught in teaching hospitals, in district general hospitals, and on attachment in GP practices. It is taught in an integrated fashion, with themes of clinical skills and communication skills running across all five years. Studying starts with the normal function of the body, building through to disease processes and clinical systems. Although there is some clinical involvement in the early years (particularly in general practice settings), the bulk of clinical placements are in years 3–5.

Teaching

The general trend is towards lectures and tutorials in the first couple of years, with formalised en-masse teaching being replaced by ward-based teaching later on in the course. Although there is some problem- or case-based work, most of the teaching is by formal lectures and small group sessions. These are balanced between tutorials and group work, with facilitators, with the aim of gaining not only knowledge but also group-work skills. Anatomy is taught with prosected material and computer-assisted learning.

Assessment

Exams have traditionally been at the end of each term and have counted for at least 60% of the course mark. There is an increasing amount of continuous and modular assessment in the new curriculum.

Intercalated degrees

At Edinburgh there is a well-established Honours year programme and a large number of students intercalate each year; you would be taking the extra year with a lot of year-group colleagues.

Special study modules and electives

Electives take place in year 5 and last for two months, and the faculty is very flexible about what you do and where you go – just as long as it's medically related. There are also several periods for special study modules (also called options, projects, etc.) starting in small groups in the first and second years and leading to an independent research project for 14 weeks in the fourth year. This is a great opportunity to do your own ground-breaking research in a university renowned for it!

Facilities

Library   There is a dedicated medical library, which is well used and is especially busy at exam times. The availability of recommended textbooks on short loan is good. It is open 9 am–10 pm Monday to Thursday, and until 5 pm on Friday and Saturday and 12–5 pm on Sunday afternoon. Holiday opening is until 7 pm, including during the summer break when there are still clinical students working. Most DGHs also have small libraries.

Computer facilities   There is a dedicated computer laboratory in the medical school with 100 PCs (and more in the medical library and throughout the university); word-processing, email, internet and specially designed computer-assisted learning are available. It is open 24 hours via a swipe card and can get very busy during the day. Many university-owned properties have computer facilities in them or on site. Facilities in hospitals outside the city are very poor, with no access to the university network, although this is set to improve.

Clinical skills   There are laboratories at both the main hospitals, which are used for learning clinical skills.

Welfare

Student support

Faculty can seem a bit harsh and traditional when you first arrive. As each student has a Director of Studies responsible for monitoring his/her progress and providing pastoral care, this effectively acts as a safety net. Faculty tends to take a hands-off approach, which on one level gives you freedom and independence, but can leave you feeling like a small drop in a big ocean. However, if you have genuine difficulties then the faculty is extremely helpful and genuinely flexible. The faculty has good relations with the Medical Students' Council and a comprehensive *Student Handbook* is published jointly every year.

Accommodation

University accommodation in halls or flats is guaranteed in the first year. However, demand from all students for halls (which are of a good standard) is greater than the places available, and after the first year most students get a group together and rent a flat from a private landlord or the university. Some students also choose to take out a mortgage to buy their own flats, renting rooms to other students. An advantage of Edinburgh is that most of the student accommodation is very central for the university and the city, and almost invariably within 15–20 minutes' walking distance. However, the cold winters do put up your heating bills.

Placements

For the first two years medics are a real part of the university, with the medical school being centrally placed in George Square. It is very handy for all the library facilities, computers, unions, and halls, as well as having the Royal Infirmary next door. The other teaching hospital is a short bus ride across town. However, the New Royal Infirmary is open now and services are gradually being moved there – several miles outside town. It is not yet clear how much of the medical school will remain on the university site and how much will move out, but it will certainly change the feel of things. In the last three years of the course most time is spent in the hospitals and often away from Edinburgh, so medics can begin to lose touch with their student roots and see less of their colleagues.

In year 1 students go into general practices twice for two well-received community-based practicals. Time in year 2 is spent in local GP practices learning clinical skills. In year 3 you may have the rare clinic outside the city. In years 4 and 5 a significant amount of time is spent on blocks in peripheral hospitals up to 80 miles from Edinburgh, as well as in general practices. There are normally at least two students on the placement, and accommodation is provided free of charge. As there are fewer students you get much more involved in the team, and the teaching is generally as good as (if not better than) in the central teaching hospitals. However, transport can be difficult if you don't have a car.

The two main teaching hospitals are the Royal Infirmary right next to the medical school, and the Western General, which is a 25-minute bus ride away (about 80p). Both have an atmosphere of pioneering, cutting-edge medicine and surgery. The facilities for students are adequate. There is a tremendous range of patients to learn from and ward groups are normally small (six or seven students in the third year – but tending to get a bit bigger – and two students per ward in the fourth and fifth years). If you put the effort in you'll get a lot out of it.

Sports and social

City life

Edinburgh, the city of festivals, is a great place to spend five years of your life. The university is centrally placed, with the medical school at the heart of the university. Although it is the capital of Scotland, Edinburgh has more than its fair share of English and overseas residents, so there is a very cosmopolitan atmosphere. For the first two years you really blend into mainstream student life, but the time-consuming clinical years mean that you gradually drift away from the main student body. There is a strong community spirit within each year group, and no shortage of medic societies, sports clubs, and socialising.

Edinburgh has the advantage of being a compact and generally safe city where everything is within walking distance. It is a lively cosmopolitan capital city with a good pub and club scene, theatres, cinemas, shopping, and a lot of tourist attractions. Although it is a huge tourist trap (especially during the Military Tattoo and the International Festival and Fringe in the summer), the tourists' and students' paths don't really cross. Between the three universities there is a large student population, which is very well catered for. Edinburgh has one of the highest concentrations of pubs in a city centre, and most are licensed to 1 am (clubs open to 3 am). Green space is found at the meadows and Holyrood Park. Both are excellent, with friendly football, rugby, hockey, American football, korfball matches, etc. Edinburgh is well connected for getting to most other parts of the UK, and the great outdoors is not too far away if you want to get away from it all for some fresh air.

Uni life

The Medical Students' Council, Royal Medical Society (which has rooms open 24 hours to members) and each year's final year club organise social events, talks, and balls. There is also a medics choir and orchestra, an active Christian Medics group, and the Medical School magazine *2nd Opinion*. In short, if you want it, it is probably there (and if it isn't you can set it up)! Apart from traditional medic activities (various balls, plays, revue, academic families), most students find their own entertainment in the city itself rather than relying exclusively upon medical societies. The Union is one of the largest in the country, offers a good range of societies, and is an excellent venue. The Unions (as a group) do have lots of competition from the city itself.

Sports life

The medics rugby team is well organised and successful, with a formidable reputation both on and off the field. A mixed hockey team and a netball team have recently been formed, and what they (sometimes) lack in skill they make up for in character. There are various year football and badminton teams. Medics tend to play a more active part in the wider university sports scene rather than just staying within the medical school. Most sports people who represent the medical school will also play for the main university and/or local clubs.

Great things about Edinburgh

- Edinburgh is a vibrant and lively university and city with excellent shopping, pubs, and clubs. The Festivals and Hogmanay are an extremely important part of the city's spirit, and the new Scottish Parliament has added to the city's cosmopolitan charms.
- Edinburgh hosts a lot of innovative and world-respected research projects in clinical medicine and surgery. You will be taught by some very big names!
- You can drink in pubs and restaurants 24 hours a day if you know how (and want to).
- Hospitals offer a good range of patients, and there is a lot of patient contact in the new course.
- The medical students have a very good collective spirit, especially in the first three years, without being too cliquey.

Bad things about Edinburgh

- Large numbers of tourists, festival luvvies and the New Year Hogmanay invasion.
- The support network works well in a crisis, but you can feel a bit anonymous to the faculty at other times.
- Peripheral attachments in the latter years mean that the year group doesn't meet up very often.
- Without a car, travelling to peripheral hospitals can be awkward.
- It gets very cold and windy in winter.

Additional application information

Average A-level requirements	• AAAB, chemistry to A-level plus maths, physics or biology. Biology at least to AS. Three A-levels accepted where verified evidence student has been unable to access four subjects
Average Scottish Higher requirements	• AAAAB, including chemistry, plus 2 out of biology, maths and physics
Make-up of interview panel	• Three members of admissions committee, all teaching staff
Months in which interviews are held	• January–March
Proportion of overseas students	• 8%
Proportion of mature students	• 3%
Faculty's view of students taking a gap year	• Happy to accept if extends general education and experience
Proportion of students taking intercalated degrees	• 40%
Possibility of direct entrance to clinical phase	• Yes, applications from only certain institutions
Fees for graduates	• See Chapter 6
Fees for overseas students	• £10 150 pa (years 1, 2) and £18 450 pa (years 3, 4, 5)
Assistance for elective funding	• Faculty gives some bursaries (up to £400 per student) and provides information on other sources
Assistance for travel to attachments	• No
Access and hardship funds	• Yes, administered centrally through the main university, and the Students Union gives short-term emergency loans
Weekly rent	• Halls £87–£94 Private £45–£60
Pint of lager	• Union bar £1.20 City centre pub £1.90
Cinema	• £3–£5
Nightclub	• Free–£12

Further information

Admissions Office
Faculty of Medicine
Medical School
Teviot Place
Edinburgh EH8 9AG
Tel: 0131 650 3187
Fax: 0131 650 6525
Email: tricia.whyte@ed.ac.uk
Web: http://www.ed.ac.uk

Glasgow

Key facts	Glasgow
Course length	5 years
Total number of medical undergraduates	c. 1200
Applicants in 2002	1327
Interviews given in 2002	49%
Places available in 2002	241
Places available in 2003	241
Entrance requirements	AAB (A-levels), AAAAB (Highers)
Mandatory subjects	Chemistry (and biology if Highers)
Male:female ratio	39:61
Premed course	No
Fast-track course	No

Glasgow is one of the longest established medical schools in Britain. In keeping with its reputation as a centre of excellence, it has radically updated its course in recent years to meet the demands of modern medicine. The new curriculum, introduced over six years ago, shifts the balance from the traditional lecture-based approach to a more problem-based method. Change and modernisation at the medical school have been matched in other areas of the university, such as a well-equipped modern library, a gym and sports complex, and a newly opened purpose-built medical school. In the unlikely event that you tire of the endless medical social functions, Glasgow has a social scene to rival that of any other major city.

Education

Glasgow radically changed its curriculum in 1996 and the course is now fully integrated, with ward teaching and clinical experience being provided from the outset. Information technology is taught and used from the first year, and the whole curriculum is student centred, with an emphasis on learning in small groups.

Teaching

Whole-class lectures only take place twice a week. The mainstay of the course is problem-based learning sessions. These involve groups of 10 students, guided by a facilitator, tackling two medical scenarios each week. The traditional preclinical/clinical divide has been significantly eroded – patient contact and practical skills are now taught from week 1.

Assessment

Continuous assessment occurs every five-week block (in first and second years) through coursework essays, and two one-hour formal written exams are taken at the end of the first year. An objective structured clinical exam (OSCE) is also part of the assessment from the second year onwards. Years 4 and 5 are treated as a continuum, with final exams only taking place at the end of the fifth year and not the fourth year.

Intercalated degrees

There are both one- and two-year intercalated degree options. One-year courses are available in clinical or science subjects and lead to a BSc MedSci (Hons). The two-year BSc (Hons) option is only available in science subjects. The intercalated degree courses are undertaken between years 3 and 4.

Special study modules and electives

Special study modules cover a wide range of subjects and constitute about 20% of the overall course time (one five-week block in year 2, and two in each year thereafter). Students choose from a list of options and may propose their own from the third year onwards. Almost any topic can be proposed, including non-medical subjects such as French or philosophy. SSMs can also be taken abroad in third, fourth, and fifth years. There are two four-week electives during the summers of the third and fourth years, which can also be spent abroad.

Facilities

Library   The main university library, with an excellent range of reference books and journals, is open until 11 pm on weekdays and during the day at weekends. The new medical school building includes a purpose-built "study landscape" well equipped with books and journals. Additional study facilities are available on campus (24 hours in Unions) and in all hospitals, some of which are open 24 hours. The new building will also have extensive library and computing facilities.

Computers   There is good central provision of computers in the main university library, with over 300 PCs available. The medical school "study landscape" provides over 100 flat-screen multimedia PCs that allow students to access a range of electronic learning facilities. Facilities are increasing and improving all the time, with about 20 PCs available for students in each of the main teaching hospitals, and peripheral hospitals gradually being linked to the campus network.

Clinical skills   Students are taught clinical skills from year 1, including first aid and basic/advanced resuscitation training. The new medical school building includes a fully equipped ward and side rooms contain audiovisual facilities to enable students to study their own performance in a simulated clinical environment before being confronted with a real hospital situation. Other new facilities include a cardiology patient simulator (known as Harvey) which can mimic symptoms of 26 cardiac diseases.

Welfare 🏠

Student support

Glasgow is renowned for its friendliness, and the medical school is no exception. Each student is allocated an Adviser of Studies to offer advice and support, and most tutors are approachable. Med-Chir (the medics' own society) operates a "Mums and Dads" scheme for freshers (with second-years acting as parents!), and Glasgow has the usual university counselling and welfare services.

Accommodation

Glasgow has a large number of students who live in the area, but it tries to guarantee accommodation to first-year students moving to the city, and 35% of hall places are reserved for returning students. The vast majority of these places are in catered halls. The university has little control over private sector flats but there is an accommodation office to help you. Average rents are £65 per week for full board in halls, £40 (plus bills) per week for a 52-week lease on a university flat, and £45–£65 (plus bills) per week for private flats.

Placements

Glasgow has a large, attractive campus in the West End of the city, two miles from the centre. Six large teaching hospitals within the Glasgow area and 13 district general hospitals (DGHs) provide the mainstay of the teaching. A new £10m medical school building, built to mark the university's 550th anniversary, was opened in September 2002. The teaching hospitals used include the Glasgow Royal Infirmary, the Western Infirmary, Gartnavel, and Stobhill Hospitals. The medical and nursing staff are approachable and friendly. Some of the DGHs used are some distance away, but accommodation is provided and the facilities are mostly OK. Groups of students number between five and eight. This drops to two per ward by the final year.

For placements outside the university, peripheral attachments can take you to Paisley (eight miles) or as far as Dumfries (65 miles). However, there are many hospitals and general practices in the Greater Glasgow area and GP practices are likely to be local.

Sports and social

City life

Glasgow is Scotland's biggest city and is truly international, with a large city centre containing all that you would expect to find. The main university buildings are among Glasgow's landmarks, with beautiful architecture and real atmosphere. The Gilbert Scott tower, the main university spire, is one of the highest points in the city. There is lots of student accommodation in flats in the West End close to the university, and near to great pubs, shops, and a lively club scene.

Glasgow was the 1999 City of Art and Design, which reflects its interesting architecture and design history. You are never short of something to do or see in Glasgow, from the well-established Kelvingrove Gallery, which houses one of the best art collections in the UK, to the new Museum of Modern Art. Glasgow also boasts some of the best shopping in Scotland (including over 40 shops in the new city centre Buchanan Galleries) and a leading club/pub scene. Not for you? How about an Old Firm game: Glasgow has the two largest Scottish football teams and many first-division rugby sides. The city hosts many international athletic events. If you want a change of scene, getting out of Glasgow is easy enough, with access to some of the best hill walking, climbing, and skiing in the UK, a mere one to two hours away. Other Scottish cities are also close at hand, with Edinburgh and the new Parliament only 45 minutes away. Buses and trains leave every 15 minutes.

Uni life

The Medico-Chirurgical Society (Med-Chir) is an educational and social society set up and run by medical students. It meets every Thursday, with free beer and talks from a range of speakers on a variety of entertaining topics. It also arranges events, including trips abroad, the annual ball, the annual revue, and a musical culture night. Each year has its own year club to organise club nights, ceilidhs, balls, and to raise money for a massive graduation ball. Our medical students' magazine *Surgo* will also keep you updated on all the activities and gossip within the faculty. Unusually, Glasgow has two Unions: Glasgow University Union (GUU) and Queen Margaret Union (QMU), both with bars, clubs, catering facilities, and a regular programme of bands, balls, and special events. The GUU has a Debating Chamber and Glasgow University has won the World Debating Championships more times than any other university. All the usual (and some unusual) clubs and societies are available for students to join (you can see a selection of them on the university website).

Sports life

The sports centre at the heart of the campus has recently undergone a massive refurbishment programme. The facilities include a 25m pool, sauna, muscle conditioning/weights room, squash courts, and sports hall. For only £20 per year you can have unlimited access to the sports facilities, as well as a wide range of daily classes in aerobics, muscle conditioning, and circuits. There are a variety of sports clubs on offer, from football and rugby through to swimming, squash, canoeing, and horse riding. Med-Chir also has medics' football and rugby teams.

Great things about Glasgow

- The new problem-based curriculum.
- West End location.
- Great facilities: two great Unions, sports complex, main library, and a well-equipped new medical school building.
- Large number of teaching hospitals.
- Teaching by internationally acclaimed experts.

Bad things about Glasgow

- The weather: Glasgow is not renowned for its sunshine.
- Some consultants are still unsure about the new curriculum.
- Some of the district hospitals are pretty far away.
- A high proportion of medics are from the Glasgow area, and this dilutes the mix of students to some extent.
- Little contact with students from other courses.

Additional application information	
Average A-level requirements	• AAB (at first attempt) in chemistry and at least one of biology, maths or physics
Average Scottish Higher requirements	• AAAAB in year 5. Chemistry and biology plus one of maths or physics
Make-up of interview panel	• Two doctors
Months in which interviews are held	• November–March
Proportion of overseas students	• 8%
Proportion of mature students	• Various by year, no quota
Faculty's view of students taking a gap year	• Acceptable as long as the year is used constructively
Proportion of students taking intercalated degrees	• 35% (mainly for one-year course)
Possibility of direct entrance to clinical phase	• No
Fees for graduates	• See Chapter 6
Fees for overseas students	• £14 700 (2002–3)
Assistance for elective funding	• Small amounts available from faculty
Weekly rent	• Halls £47–£49 (self-catered and catered) Private £45–£65
Pint of lager	• Union bar £1.50 City centre pub £2.20
Cinema	• £2.50–£4.90
Nightclub	• Free–£15

Further information

Admissions Enquiries
Wolfson Medical School
University of Glasgow
University Avenue
Glasgow G128QQ
Tel: 0141 330 6216
Fax: 0141 330 2776
Email: amp1v@clinmed.gla.ac.uk
Web: http://www.medicine.gla.ac.uk

Guy's, King's and St Thomas'

Key facts	GRT
Course length	5 years
Total number of medical undergraduates	1800
Applicants in 2002	3020
Interviews given in 2002	40% – no place is offered without interview
Places available in 2002	360
Places available in 2003	360
Entrance requirements	ABB
Mandatory subjects	Chemistry and biology (at least one to A-level)
Male:female ratio	39:61
Premed course	Yes
Fast-track course	Yes for suitably qualified BOS/MFOS graduates

Guy's, King's and St Thomas' School of Medicine, popularly known as GKT, was formed in August 1998 by the merger of the United Medical and Dental School (UMDS) of Guy's and St Thomas' Hospitals and King's College School of Medicine and Dentistry (KCSMD) to form part of King's College London. The first joint intake started in 1999 and has so far gone well.

The school combines two established medical schools, both with long histories, including older mergers. King's College is a multidisciplinary institution, part of the University of London, and had its own medical school at King's College Hospital in south London. Guy's and St Thomas' Hospitals had their own medical schools prior to the 1992 merger to form the United Medical and Dental Schools.

An intake of over 360 students makes the new school one of the biggest medical schools in the UK, and King's College as a whole the largest centre for healthcare teaching in Europe. Both King's and UMDS emphasised personal academic development (for example a strongly supported intercalated BSc programme) and encouraged students to participate fully in extracurricular activities. This is a strong feature of the new GKT.

Education

The course is split into two main sections. The first two years place an emphasis on the basic medical sciences. There is early clinical contact, with communication teaching taking place in a GP setting from the first year. The course is organised into systems, for example cardiovascular or musculoskeletal. The majority of students appear to find this a more useful way of learning. A disadvantage, however, is that many textbooks concentrate on specific subject areas, such as biochemistry or anatomy, and it is sometimes necessary to look at up to four books at the same time when studying. All the core basic science teaching takes place at the Guy's Hospital campus.

Clinical disciplines are taught in the latter three years on the wards of St Thomas' Hospital, King's College Hospital, Guy's Hospital, University Hospital Lewisham, and also in the community. A new systems-based clinical course has been designed and was introduced in 1988 to complement the course structure from the earlier years. The core clinical subjects are delivered and examined during years 3 and 4. The final year consists of an eight-week elective, followed by attachments in the community and attachments shadowing house officers in district general hospitals.

Teaching

There is a mixture of lectures, tutorials, and practicals, mixed in with computer-assisted learning. Dissection is still seen as a valued part of preclinical teaching.

Assessment

Essay and short-answer questions are now rare during years 3–5. Written examinations during the clinical years are now mostly computer marked, and offer some element of choice in the answer. Negative marking for wrong answers in MCQ exams has been abolished. OSCEs (objective structured clinical exams) are the main practical examinations during the clinical years, starting with a short communication skills OSCE in year 2.

Intercalated degrees

There are well-supported intercalated degree programmes at the college. There is a wide range of options to choose from, including many outside medicine and the sciences, sometimes even at other London colleges.

Special study modules and electives

About 20% of each year is devoted to SSMs. There is a considerable range of subjects available and the number is increasing every year. As the school is part of a multifaculty institution there are also many non-medical SSMs available, such as a choice of modern languages and the popular history of medicine. Students may also design their own SSMs if the subject they wish to study is not on offer.

The eight-week elective period is an opportunity to travel to far-flung destinations (or just down the road) to study in fields of medicine of your choosing. There is some assessment of how time is spent on the elective (to discourage the temptation to just lie on a beach for 12 weeks), and at the moment this is in the form of a poster presentation. Various awards and sponsorships are available to help students fund their electives. The school has special links with numerous medical schools around the world, including the Johns Hopkins University in the USA, the University of Hong Kong, the University of West Indies, and Moscow Medical Academy. As GKT is twinned with these institutions, there are special allocations for GKT students who want to do their electives there. Accommodation will also usually be arranged for you, and extra bursaries may be available to help with travel costs to these colleges.

Added opportunities

Access to medicine is a major initiative to widen access to medical degree courses. Last year GKT launched a programme specifically designed to help bright and talented young people from disadvantaged backgrounds to become doctors. The programme will eventually allow for up to 50 extra undergraduate places in medicine and will be for talented school pupils from south London who would not normally achieve the necessary grades to train as doctors. The course is based on a standard MBBS course but will take six years rather than five, because of the addition of special modules in the first three years.

Facilities

Library Libraries at Guy's are open between 9 am and 8.45 pm on weekdays, 9 am and 4.45 pm on Saturday, and 1 pm and 4.45 pm on Sunday; there is also a large 24-hour study room. At King's College Hospital the library is open until 9 pm on weekdays and 1 pm on Saturday. Students also have access to the King's College London library at the old Public Records Office on Chancery Lane, which is open until 9 pm from Monday to Thursday, 6 pm on Friday, and 5.30 pm on Saturday. All libraries have a good range of books and journals.

Computers All campuses have a large number of computer stations with access to email, the internet, and computer-assisted learning programs designed in-house. There are 24-hour computing facilities at Guy's, and late/weekend opening at the St Thomas' campus. The "virtual campus" is a specialised area of the King's College London website for the GKT Schools of Medicine, Dentistry and Biomedical Sciences and enables students to do things like download lecture notes, register for course components, or obtain details (but not the answers) about their exams.

Clinical skills A new clinical skills centre opened at Guy's in 1999. It is the largest of its kind in Europe, and is available every weekday from 9 am to 5 pm. Students can book individual rooms in small groups or with their tutor. There are also various laboratories at the three main hospitals. These are great places, with latex models of every imaginable part of the human anatomy on which students can practise their clinical skills, such as taking blood pressure or suturing (in the past, King's students on accident and emergency attachments practised suturing pigs' trotters before being let loose on the population of south London!).

Welfare

Student support

Students are assigned to a personal tutor to support them throughout the course. Welfare and counselling services are available on the Guy's campus, where there is a welfare officer available every day. All sites are friendly environments with lots of support from the faculty and staff. The Student Medical Education Committee (SMEC) is a unique student committee that is actively involved in course development and provides feedback to course organisers on how things are going. It acts as a dedicated link between the medical school and the student body. There are six elected representatives in each year, and they will help students to deal with any problems that arise with the course and address any associated welfare concerns.

Accommodation

College accommodation is available in many different parts of London. Some residences may be on or near the campuses themselves (on-site accommodation is available on the Guy's campus), whereas others may be much further away. The quality and cost of private accommodation can vary a lot in the central Guy's/St Thomas' area, but cheaper, good-quality accommodation is more readily available in the Denmark Hill area. Students can opt for Intercollegiate University of London accommodation, although these tend to be some distance from any of the campuses.

Placements

Students in years 1 and 2 are taught at the newly developed Guy's Hospital campus at London Bridge. The campus is shared with other departments in the biomedical sciences and dentistry. Most of the Guy's site has been refurbished to accommodate the large number of students, and many facilities are new. A large new building houses most of the above disciplines, with state-of-the-art library and computing facilities. Most of the clinical teaching takes place at St Thomas' Hospital, King's College Hospital, Guy's Hospital, and University Hospital Lewisham. Students can also access King's College's other campuses, including the Strand campus and Waterloo. Guy's, St Thomas', and the Strand campuses are all situated within a square mile on both sides of the Thames in central London. Psychiatry teaching happens at the Maudsley Hospital and other institutions in south London.

As well as the central teaching hospitals in years 4 and 5, there are placements in district general hospitals in southeast England. This relieves some of the pressures at the central London teaching hospitals and provides access to high-quality teaching; clinical workloads tend to be lower, and consultants are able to devote more time to students.

Sports and social 🏆

City life

Most of the campuses are close to the centre of London, with all of London's attractions within easy reach by public transport.

Uni life

The old colleges always had thriving social scenes, with numerous balls, weekly hops, the annual revues, and rag week. The traditions have all continued after the merger, and as the college grows more exciting developments are expected. There is a vast selection of clubs and societies to join, and everyone can usually find something that interests them. The Student Union is based on the Guy's campus, where a new nightclub and bar were built in 1999. Student bars are present on all campuses, and there is the main college nightclub at the Strand campus. If all that's not enough, all students have access to the University of London Union (ULU) with its own range of facilities.

GKT gives students access to a large multidisciplinary institution while retaining the friendliness of a medical school. With its almost enclosed courtyard, promenade, and grass park at London Bridge, the Guy's campus is regarded as the closest thing to a campus university in central London. The mix of students on a day-to-day basis may not be diverse, but as students use King's College and University of London Union facilities there will be plenty of opportunity for integration.

Sports life

Particularly strong sports include rugby, football, hockey, netball, tennis, badminton, rowing, and squash, alongside the oldest rugby team in the world at Guy's. GKT has sports grounds at Honor Oak Park in south London, Dulwich, and Cobham in Surrey, giving facilities for rugby, football, and hockey. King's College also has sports grounds in Surbiton. There are gyms at the Guy's and St Thomas' campuses, and also at the Stamford Street halls of residence. For swimmers, there is a pool at Guy's.

Great things about GKT

- GKT hospitals are all world renowned.
- Excellent range of learning and social facilities at the medical school campuses, with more on the way.
- The new school is part of a multifaculty institution. Students will have the opportunity to mix with a variety of students from other courses, and have access to a wide range of facilities.
- Good sports clubs (some with lots of history).
- Welfare and student support mechanisms are well established and are effective.

Bad things about GKT

- Cost of living in London.
- Student accommodation can be a long way from your campus.
- Large number of medics in each year group can lead to it being a bit impersonal.
- Split-site arrangements leads to some inconvenience when moving around.
- The medical school can be a bit bureaucratic.

Additional application information	
Average A-level requirements	• AAB (at first attempt) in chemistry and at least one of biology, maths or physics
Average Scottish Higher requirements	• AAAAB in year 5. Chemistry and biology plus one of maths or physics
Make-up of interview panel	• Two doctors
Months in which interviews are held	• November-March
Proportion of overseas students	• 8%
Proportion of mature students	• Various by year, no quota
Faculty's view of students taking a gap year	• Acceptable as long as the year is used constructively
Proportion of students taking intercalated degrees	• 35% (mainly for one-year course)
Possibility of direct entrance to clinical phase	• No
Fees for graduates	• See Chapter 6
Fees for overseas students	• £14 700 (2002–3)
Assistance for elective funding	• Small amounts available from faculty
Weekly rent	• Halls £47–£49 (self-catered and catered) Private £45–£65
Pint of lager	• Union bar £1.50 City centre pub £2.20
Cinema	• £2.50–£4.90
Nightclub	• Free–£15

Further information

Student Admissions Officer
The Hodgkin Building
Guy's Hospital Campus
King's College London
St Thomas' Street
London Bridge
London SE1 9RT
Tel: 020 7848 6501/6502
Fax: 020 7848 6510
Email: gktadmissions@kcl.ac.uk
Web: http://www.kcl.ac.uk

Hull York

Key facts	Hull
Course length	5 years
Total number of medical undergraduates	650 proposed (130 per annum)
Applicants in 2002	-
Interviews given in 2002	-
Places available in 2002	-
Places available in 2003	130
Entrance requirements	ABB or equivalent (A2) for school leavers
Mandatory subjects	Biology and chemistry
Male:female ratio	-
Premed course	No
Fast-track course	No

Opening in 2003

The Universities of Hull and York made a successful bid to share a new medical school to accommodate the expanding number of medical student places in the UK. We cannot give you an *Insiders' Guide* to the new medical school because the first students will begin their studies in September 2003. The following is a statement from the School.

HYMS (the Hull York Medical School) is a new medical school, which will award joint degrees from the long-established and well-respected universities of Hull and York. Both have considerable experience in medical and bioscience education. The University of Hull has 10 years' experience of medicine through its postgraduate medical school, with strong research activity in cardiovascular and respiratory medicine, gastrointestinal and cancer surgery, and oncology. The University of York's bioscience and health science departments are highly rated for both teaching and research, and together the universities provide an enviable academic base for HYMS.

The HYMS course aims to make medical education exciting and effective: modern methods of problem-based learning, computer-aided learning, and a fully integrated five-year curriculum will put HYMS at the cutting edge of medical education. In addition, an optional extra year may be offered to

105

selected students to complete a science Honours degree (BSc) in a subject of their choice, from the many specialist courses offered on both universities.

In years 1 and 2, students will study basic sciences in the context of clinical medicine in every system block. Small groups of students will meet patients with relevant medical problems who will explain both their symptoms and the psychological and social impact of their illness. In this way you will find it easier to make sense of the complex biological information essential for a sound foundation in medicine. In years 3 and 4 the course becomes truly multicentred, with teaching in centres across north and east Yorkshire and northern Lincolnshire. With accommodation on hospital sites and linked general practice attachments, students will benefit from low student–teacher ratios, and plenty of opportunities for hands-on learning in both hospital and primary care. The final year comprises three substantial blocks of study in medicine, surgery, and general practice, and an elective period bridging the fourth and final years.

Assessments will be carefully designed to address the outcomes of each stage of the course, and will use a combination of factual tests and practical patient-based assessments.

Students will be based in either Hull or York for the first two years of the degree and will be offered university accommodation. In years 3, 4, and 5 the Hull and York groups will combine, and together follow a programme of community- and hospital-based study in centres throughout east and north Yorkshire and north Lincolnshire. Accommodation when away from Hull or York will normally be in NHS facilities. In this way you will gain a wide experience of medicine in both specialist and generalist practice.

On successful completion, students will receive a joint medical degree from the Universities of Hull and York, which will be recognised by the General Medical Council and allow practice as a preregistration house officer in a recognised supervised post. HYMS will continue to be responsible for your training and development throughout this year. Most of these posts are in hospital, but it will be possible to spend some of the year in general practice.

HYMS expects applicants to have achieved high grades across a broad range of subjects at GCSE, and to show evidence of breadth in sixth form studies. We shall expect three A-levels (apart from general studies) at grades ABB, including chemistry and biology at A-level. Some experience of caring for others is an advantage, but can be evidenced in a variety of ways. Interpersonal skills are also important, and an interview is expected to be a normal part of the selection process.

Additional application information

Average A-level requirements	• ABB, including biology and chemistry
Average Scottish Higher requirements	• Grades AABBB, including biology and chemistry
Make-up of interview panel	• Two people, one of whom will be a health professional
Months in which interviews are held	• December–February
Proportion of overseas students	• None
Proportion of mature students	• Up to 15%
Faculty's view of students taking a gap year	• Positive in the right circumstances
Proportion of students taking intercalated degrees	• Up to 15%
Possibility of direct entrance to clinical phase	• Not possible

Further information

Student Recruitment and Admissions Service
University of Hull
Kingston upon Hull
Hull HU6 7RX
Tel: 01482 46100
Email: admissions@hull.ac.uk

Admissions and Schools Liaison
University of York
Heslington
York Y010 5DD
Tel: 01904 433533
Email: admissions@york.ac.uk
Web: http://www.hyms.ac.uk, http://www.hull.ac.uk

Imperial College London

Key facts	Imperial
Course length	6 years
Total number of medical undergraduates	c. 2000
Applicants in 2002	2500
Interviews given in 2002	41%
Places available in 2002	326
Places available in 2003	326
Entrance requirements	ABB + A at AS-level
Mandatory subjects	Chemistry and biology
Male:female ratio	44:56
Premed course	No
Fast-track course	No

Imperial College Faculty of Medicine is the product of a merger between Charing Cross and Westminster, and St Mary's Schools of Medicine. The first intake on the new course began in autumn 1998. By 2003 there will be no students from the original medical schools: all will be of the combined Imperial entry. Imperial College School of Medicine has created a new identity while maintaining the spirit and traditions of the original schools. Initial teething problems created by the merger and the new course have been resolved. Research at both medical schools has traditionally been strong, and this has been aided by incorporation into Imperial College. There is a new building (the Sir Alexander Fleming building) at the Imperial College site in South Kensington, which is very central and only 200m from Hyde Park. All first-year halls of residence are close to this site. Imperial is now one of the largest medical schools in the country, and the non-course elements such as sport and music are flourishing in their new environment.

Education

Imperial offers a six-year course which incorporates an intercalated Honours year for everyone except appropriately qualified graduates, who may apply for an exemption. Non-graduate mature students are expected to undertake six years. There is integrated teaching from day 1, which includes early ward exposure and general practice experience. There is a term-based structure for the first and second years (see prospectus). A wide variety of clinical experience is offered, at many sites. The course takes advantage of the large number of hospitals in west London. New courses have been introduced, including a business course and an introduction to graduate medical practice. The integrated course has now matured and adapted to the comments of the pioneering students. This has made it a well-tailored and enjoyable one. Everyone has been keen to make Imperial a success and there is a genuine willingness to adapt and improve components.

Teaching

A mixture of exams and continuous assessment is used to monitor students' progress. Problem-based learning in small groups is a key feature of the teaching at Imperial, but lectures remain the mainstay of teaching. Students are encouraged to use computers and clinical skills laboratories. Lectures and ward attachments occur during all parts of the course, but as you progress more time is spent in hospital attachments. Anatomy is taught from the second year by dissection of cadavers. However, most anatomy teaching uses predissected models.

Assessment

End-of-year exams form the basis of assessment in the first three years, with more regular assessments after most firms as you progress into the clinical years. Retakes are offered after all end-of-year exams if things don't go to plan. They are traditionally held in the September before the following academic year. Vivas have been phased out at Imperial, which many students have welcomed. As a BSc is a compulsory inclusion to the Imperial course this is assessed at the end of the year in a terminal exam, throughout the year via essays, and finally on the project.

Intercalated degrees

A compulsory BSc has been built into the new course which is normally undertaken in years 4 or 5, although some modules are undertaken from year 2. The BSc is a modular degree programme and there is a wide range of subject choices, for example genetics, psychology, biochemistry, and management (taught at the Imperial College Management School alongside MBA students).

Special study modules and electives

There is a 12-week elective in year 6 where you are encouraged to learn and explore how medicine is practised abroad. Imperial College offers many grants each year to students undertaking valuable study abroad, which helps ease the cost. SSMs in the final year cover four two-week courses in subjects of your choice. There is a wide range of specialties to choose from, ranging from alternative medicine to radiology.

Facilities

Library There are libraries at all sites, which are open from 9 am till 9 pm on weekdays and also on Saturday mornings. They do hold reference copies of all recommended texts, but loan copies generally disappear quite quickly. All libraries also hold videos of clinical lectures, so that if you miss one or don't understand one, you can always review it at your leisure – you can't always make every 9 am!

Computers There is a considerable emphasis on IT in the Imperial course. To sustain this, the number of computer facilities is expanding considerably, and training is also provided. The Charing Cross campus has recently installed new machines, some with CD writers. There are computer facilities for Imperial College medical students at all peripheral attachments.

Clinical skills These are at Charing Cross and St Mary's hospitals and at some peripheral hospitals too. Students are encouraged to use them as part of their training in both timetabled and student-arranged sessions. They are very well equipped and good fun to use. You can practise everything from taking blood to doing a rectal examination on latex dummies. These help you build confidence before doing procedures on real patients.

Welfare

Student support

The 2003/4 entry will be the first year where all students at Imperial College will be of the merged schools. This has the advantage that there will be five batches of students in years above who have done the same course. This puts them in the best place to advise you. Students in the first years, who are based at South Kensington, can feel remote from the medical environment. Soon after starting at Imperial, each fresher is allocated a "parent" student (of the opposite sex) from the year above. "Parents" are able to help you adjust to university and medical school life. They also help you to ease in to the social life and can offer advice and tips about the course; they will probably even cook you dinner and show you why medic life is so renowned. Each student is also allocated a tutor, who should be available for personal and academic problems and advice. However, the reality is that some students may go through six years without ever meeting him/her. Imperial College has counselling and welfare services available to all students.

Accommodation

First-years have a guaranteed place in halls at about £85 per week. Halls are 2–30 minutes from one of the three main hospitals, and no more than an hour from all the peripheral sites. Private sector accommodation is expensive if you want to live near to Imperial College in South Kensington (£85–£100+ per week). However, as you will spend the majority of your time from your second year onwards based in the Hammersmith hospitals, most students live in and around Hammersmith where rent is less expensive – £75–£95.

Placements

The school uses a wide range of centres across central and west London for teaching. The main teaching hospitals – Charing Cross (Hammersmith), Chelsea and Westminster (Fulham), and St Mary's (Paddington) – are supplemented by peripheral district general hospitals and teaching hospitals in Middlesex and Surrey. A new building (the Sir Alexander Fleming building) at the main Imperial College site is used for basic biomedical sciences, which constitutes much of the first year. There are adequate public transport links between all sites, and a London Transport discount scheme has reduced the travel costs.

Students experience a wide range of clinical attachments, starting with a GP practice placement in the first year. Initially many attachments will be near to Imperial College, but as you proceed into your specialist clinical studies (years 4–6) they may be further afield (outside London), but you are generally offered a shortlist of hospitals to choose from. Free hospital accommodation is nearly always provided if needed.

Sports and social

City life

Nothing written in a small paragraph could do justice to the multitude of activities, events, venues, clubs, and locations that London offers. Suffice to say that if you went to a different restaurant, cinema, ice rink, museum, or club each day for the six years you are here, there would still be more to see!

Uni life

The medical school has made a name for itself by incorporating the best of both its parent schools. The central London setting and the wide range of people have assisted this process. Opportunities for non-medical pursuits abound, but the traditional medical student lifestyle is in no danger of disappearing. The medical school's own Students' Union and societies help Imperial medics maintain a separate identity from the rest of Imperial College students. However, medical students can also take advantage of Imperial College Union and its teams and clubs. There is a newly refurbished £1m student bar at the Charing Cross campus, which holds regular events (however, no-one seems to know how to turn the air conditioning on!). Highlights of the year include fresher's roadshow, the interyear rugby match, rag week, including the Circle line pub crawl, and the summer ball. There are plenty of medical student events spread through each term organised by either the medical school union or individual clubs and societies.

Sports life

Imperial College medical school teams have grounds at Teddington (previously home to England RFC) and Cobham, and Imperial College has pitches and an Astroturf at Gunnersbury. Students can also use one of three Imperial College-owned sports centres. The Imperial medics rugby team (old boys including J.P.R. Williams) has already made a name for itself at a European level, and the school frequently holds many United Hospitals trophies. A substantial rugby scholarship is also awarded annually to the fresher who has made the greatest impression at the club. Rowing at Imperial College is world class and training facilities reflect this. Women's sports are well established, with hockey and netball being among the most popular. The men's cricket team pride themselves on their post-match celebrations. Other sports include water polo, mountaineering, surfing, and mixed lacrosse, to name but a few. The variety of sporting choice is paralleled only by the mixture of abilities: from the social players to the semiprofessionals and internationals, all are welcome and encouraged.

Great things about Imperial

- The opportunities available here will ensure you leave with the greatest of experiences.
- State-of-the-art audiovisual system, meaning that if you are at one site and the lecture is at another it can be beamed to your site; this reduces the need to travel and hence cost.
- You can choose between the close-knit medical community at the medical school, the larger Imperial College environment, or metropolitan city life.
- A brand new building for biomedical sciences, at the South Kensington Imperial College site, as well as Chelsea and Westminster Hospital (known as the "Hilton Hospital") means salubrious surroundings.
- Large city with a huge range of cultural activities – anything you want can be found.

Bad things about Imperial

- 2002 intake was so large there is no lecture theatre big enough to hold the whole year.
- Travel between sites adds to the expense of studying and can be stressful.
- Split teaching hospital sites divides the year groups up.
- Imperial College is sometimes pictured as boring and academic. But remember that's NOT the medics!
- Expensive, polluted, overpopulated, time-consuming, dirty old London, etc.

Additional application information

Average A-level requirements	• ABB plus grade A in fourth AS subject. Chemistry and biology to AS-level. Chemistry or biology to A-level
Average Scottish Higher requirements	• Not acceptable unless offered in conjunction with Advanced Highers, CSYS or A-levels (contact admissions office for advice on subjects)
Make-up of interview panel	• Chair, external clinician, academic, and clinical student
Months in which interviews are held	• November–April
Proportion of overseas students	• 7%
Proportion of mature students	• 2.5%
Faculty's view of students taking a gap year	• Encouraged for students using the year constructively
Proportion of students taking intercalated degrees	• Intercalated degree built into the course
Possibility of direct entrance to clinical phase	• Oxbridge only
Fees for graduates	• £1100
Fees for overseas students	• £12 250 pa (preclinical) and £20 700 pa (clinical)
Assistance for elective funding	• Three scholarships from three trusts
Assistance for travel to attachments	• None from university
Access and hardship funds	• Yes (students in final years tend to be more successful)
Weekly rent	• Halls £60–£84 Private £75–£110
Pint of lager	• Union bar £1.50 City centre pub £2.30
Cinema	• £3.50–£8
Nightclub	• Free–£20

Further information

School of Medicine
Imperial College
London SW7 2AZ
Tel: 020 7589 5111
Fax: 020 7594 8004
Email: admitmed@ic.ac.uk
Web: http://www.med.ic.uk

Leeds

Key facts	Leeds
Course length	5 years
Total number of medical undergraduates	1100
Applicants in 2002	1839
Interviews given in 2002	34%
Places available in 2002	238
Places available in 2003	223
Entrance requirements	AAB
Mandatory subjects	Chemistry
Male:female ratio	40:60
Premed course	No
Fast-track course	No

The course at Leeds has undergone several changes recently and there is now a new integrated curriculum: out with the old subject-based teaching of anatomy, biochemistry, physiology, etc. and in with a module-based integrated course. There is some clinically oriented teaching from year 1, and hospital-based teaching starts towards the end of year 2. Staff and departments have been receptive to any balanced criticisms and suggestions, and this has generated a student-friendly atmosphere. The medical school has a real mix of students from up and down the country, as well as overseas and mature students. Medics here sometimes feel a little separated from the rest of the student population, but they get a chance to mix in halls of residence and sports clubs. A strong feeling of togetherness within and between year groups, and a good Medsoc and Medical Students' Representative Committee (MSRC) make up for this.

Education

The course is systems based, including clinical experience from year 1. Modules include personal and professional development, biomedical sciences, transport, life cycles, nutrition and energy, and control and movement. For years 1 and 2 the academic year follows the rest of the university, but from year 3 it becomes longer at the expense of holidays. New GMC guidelines have also reduced the number of exams in years 1 and 2.

Teaching

Teaching is integrated, with a mix of problem-solving exercises, small group teaching, and lectures. The use of computer-based learning is increasing rapidly, with experiments, tutorials, and practice test questions being placed on computer. Anatomy is still taught using dissection of human cadavers. Ward teaching begins in the second year.

Assessment

Assessments include essays, projects, and both essay and multiple choice exams.

Intercalated degrees

A year-long BSc can be taken, usually after the second or third year. The number of students intercalating has increased sharply in recent years to approximately 40–50%, and there is a range of scholarships available.

Special study modules and electives

A 10-week elective is timetabled at the beginning of the fifth year. Many students travel overseas for this, and recent destinations have been Canada, Australia, Africa, and Barbados. Special study modules start in the first year and make up a substantial part of the course.

Facilities

Library   The medical library is well equipped and stocked, and is open until 9 pm Monday to Thursday, 7 pm on Friday and 5 pm on Saturday.

Computers   There is very good provision of computers throughout Leeds University, with 200 in the medical school and about 50 in a cluster at St James' Hospital (Jimmy's). There is an IT course at the beginning of the first year to help improve computer literacy.

Clinical skills   There are clinical skills laboratories at St James' Hospital and at Leeds General Infirmary (LGI).

Welfare

Student support

Levels of support at Leeds are generally good. The MUMS scheme has been running for a number of years and enables students from different years to interact with first-years to provide pastoral care. The Students Union and the university have counselling services.

Accommodation

All first-years can live in university accommodation, either halls or flats. These can be pricey, but standards are generally good and this can be a good way to meet non-medics. In the second year most move out to back-to-back houses in Leeds 6 – Studentsville. Rents start at about £45 per week, but most pay a little more. Insurance is pricey, and burglary can be a problem. The locals can sometimes be a little anti-student, but your mates all live in the next street. There is help in finding accommodation available from the university.

Placements

The medical school lies on the very edge of Leeds University campus and is attached to the Leeds General Infirmary (one of the main teaching hospitals). The city centre is a 10-minute walk from the school, and buses run from the campus to all parts of Leeds. Facilities in the teaching hospitals are generally OK. Lots of teaching happens at the two main Leeds hospitals – Jimmy's and the LGI. A lot of district general hospitals are used, including York, Harrogate, Ilkley, Halifax, Scunthorpe, Otley, Bradford, Hull, Huddersfield, and Wakefield. A few third-year students spend a term in the Yorkshire Dales. In the fourth and fifth years attachments can be even further afield. All accommodation and transport is provided for residential attachments. Travel costs are variable and are to a degree supported by the university. Leeds medical school district hospitals incorporate the majority of West and North Yorkshire, with Sheffield medical school serving South Yorkshire. It depends where you live in Leeds, but the furthest you may have to travel is Hull (about 61 ± 3 miles), which can take well over an hour in rush-hour traffic.

Sports and social 🏆

City life

Leeds is the fastest-growing city in the UK outside London. The main city centre has all the shopping and nightlife your bank account can take, within a 10–15-minute walk from campus. Theatre, Opera North, museums, and galleries cater for the culture vultures. Sport is big in Leeds, especially football, cricket, and rugby league.

"Possibly the shopping capital of the north!" The city centre boasts the first Harvey Nichols outside London, and with the many other shops there is everything anyone could want. The Yorkshire Dales are a short bus journey away and a fantastic place to walk and get away from the hustle and bustle of life in Leeds. There are good road links and Leeds is on the Intercity rail network.

Uni life

The Union has four bars, including the biggest in Europe (allegedly). Medsoc is probably the most active society of the Union and organises endless events, including two annual balls, pub crawls, ice-skating, quizzes, ballet trips, and lots of general drinking nights – something for everyone. The university also has a wide range of clubs and societies.

Sports life

Medics' rugby, football, hockey, netball, cricket, and racket games are all supported by MSRC. The university has a large sports centre, loads of gym equipment, aerobics classes, yoga, kickboxing, etc. The main university runs many sports teams as well.

Great things about Leeds

- The friendliness among medics between different years.
- The Leeds nightlife means there is always something for everyone to do.
- Very active medical student committees organising everything from balls to sports events.
- Proximity to the Dales – a city in the country!
- Leeds is a city on the up and there is a definite buzz about the centre (and fantastic shopping), with an impressive new Millennium Square.

Bad things about Leeds

- There are so many distractions from studying.
- Medics always seem to have exams and assessments when the rest of the university hasn't, and vice versa.
- Increased use of computers can lead to problems of access.
- Traffic, particularly at rush hour, and lots of road works are choking the city centre.
- Everywhere in Leeds is hilly!

Additional application information

Average A-level requirements	• AAB at A-level or AB (plus AA at AS-level.) A-level chemistry. General studies not accepted
Average Scottish Higher requirements	• AAAAB at higher level with BB at CSYS/Advanced Higher level (chemistry required)
Make-up of interview panel	• Two consultants plus one medical student
Months in which interviews are held	• December–March
Proportion of overseas students	• Quota of 15 places per year
Proportion of mature students	• 6%
Faculty's view of students taking a gap year	• Positive if the year is used for work experience, voluntary service or travel
Proportion of students taking intercalated degrees	• 40–50%
Possibility of direct entrance to clinical phase	• Because of integrated curriculum there is no longer a preclinical or clinical year, transfers are difficult to arrange and would only be considered when there are extenuating circumstances and strong support from the host medical school
Fees for graduates	• Subject to change. Check with university
Fees for overseas students	• £17 768 (but subject to change. Check with university)
Assistance for elective funding	• Various awards and prizes available
Assistance for travel to attachments	• Third-year travel provided, some reimbursement for costs in years 4 and 5
Access and hardship funds	• Access funds from Leeds University
Weekly rent	• Halls £40–£93 Private £45–£55
Pint of lager	• Union bar £1.30 City centre pub £2.10
Cinema	• £2–£5
Nightclub	• £3–£10

Further information

Admissions Office
School of Medicine
University of Leeds
Leeds LS2 9JT
Tel: 0113 233 4362
Fax: 0113 233 4375
Email: prospectus@leeds.ac.uk
Web: http://www.leeds.ac.uk

Leicester/Warwick

Key facts	Leicester	Warwick graduate entry	Leicester graduate entry
Course length	5 years	4 years	4 years
Total number of medical students	908	331	N/A
Applicants in 2002	1400	800	N/A
Interviews given in 2002	60%		N/A
Places available in 2002	175	128	N/A
Places available in 2003	175	164	64
Entrance requirements	AAB	2:1 degree	2:1 degree
Mandatory subjects	Chemistry A2 Biology AS	Biomedical science degree	Health studies/ Health sciences
Male:female ratio	45:55	40:60	N/A
Premed course	No	No	No
Fast-track course	No	Yes	Yes

Leicester is a young medical school whose first students graduated in 1980. It is a friendly place, with the teaching for Phase I being on the university campus, which is next to Victoria Park about 10–15 minutes' walk from the city centre. Most of the main halls are further out in one of the nicer areas of Leicester and they have beautiful gardens. The later phases of the course are based mainly at the Clinical Sciences Building (CSB). This is part of Leicester Royal Infirmary and near the city centre. The Union provides many a good night out, and there is also a wide range of nights out and other events organised by MedSoc, including balls, outings, and skiing trips.

The Universities of Leicester and Warwick joined up in 2000 to offer an accelerated four-year medical degree course to graduates in biomedical sciences. The course started with 64 students and the first intake began their studies at Warwick on an accelerated version of Phase I of the Leicester five-year degree programme. Upon successful completion of Phase I students join with the Phase II programme at the University of Leicester. The joining of the two universities gives further emphasis to Leicester's reputation as an innovative and youthful medical school.

Education

Leicester In common with most other medical schools, Leicester has largely done away with the traditional preclinical/clinical divide. The course is now separated into two phases, each lasting

2½ years. Phase I is taught in the Medical Sciences Building (MSB) and is based on tutorials and lectures. There is, however, an introduction to clinical skills and you are let loose on wards in November of the second year. Anatomy is taught using dissection and prosections. There is also a clinical applications module to be completed in the third year on a disease of your choice. Phase II is mainly clinical, with ward teaching in different specialties, and includes an elective period. Progression between the two phases is subject to passing examinations.

Warwick Students on the four-year graduate-entry course complete Phase I at Warwick. Phase I is modular, with modules covering mechanisms of disease, health policy issues, and understanding the skills and knowledge needed to be a doctor. Team working is emphasised. There is clinical content during this phase and body systems are studied in an integrated way (studying anatomy, biochemistry, physiology, etc. all at the same time).

Teaching

Leicester For Phase I teaching you are placed in a group of eight for tutorial work and will remain with this group throughout the phase. Examinations are mainly written short-answer questions or assessed essays.

Phase II teaching is on the wards, but it is backed by some lectures (an academic half-day per week). You will be with a clinical partner of your choice. Attendance is registered and contributes to passing modules. There are 13 eight-week blocks, which rotate through disciplines and include an elective. For each block, the pair of clinical students is attached to two consultant teams, one from a subspecialty and one more general. Assessment includes patient portfolios (case studies) and clinical skills (histories and examinations). Finals have a clinical component and written examinations.

Warwick During Phase I students travel to Leicester for anatomy sessions (not really a placement). Hospitals and general practices used during the first three semesters are all in the Coventry area. In Phase II (clinical phase), the Warwick site uses all the same hospital rotations as the Leicester site.

Assessment

Warwick During Phase I students on the four-year course are assessed in a way that allows for quality assurance with the five-year course. This includes MCQ and short-answer questions.

Intercalated degrees

Leicester Any student wishing to do an Honours year is encouraged to do so. Honours degrees can be science based or clinical and there is a wide range of projects to choose from. The degree is usually taken after the second year, but can be done after the third.

Warwick All students are graduates and intercalated degrees are not offered.

Special study modules and electives

Leicester All students have a two-month elective module which can be carried out in the UK or abroad. Two special study modules (SSM) are done in Phase I, and one in Phase II. It is compulsory to study one science SSM, although other subjects such as languages are available as the second. Furthermore, there is an opportunity in the third year to spend 10 weeks on a short Erasmus exchange to Germany, Spain, or Switzerland.

Warwick There are two SSMs within Phase I of the Warwick course.

Facilities

Library
Leicester The main university library is on campus and near to the MSB. There are also libraries at the three main teaching hospitals, but the CSB library at the Leicester Royal Infirmary is the main library used by medical students. The MSB and CSB libraries open from 9 am to 10 pm on weekdays. The hours are shorter on Saturday (9 am–6 pm) and Sunday (12 pm–9 pm).

Warwick Warwick has a huge library on the central campus. This is well generally resourced, but time will be needed to build up the core of medical knowledge to more satisfactory levels.

Computers
Leicester There are computer facilities in the main library, Charles Wilson, Kenneth Edward, and MSB on the main campus, but you do have to queue sometimes. There are plenty of computers (mostly PCs) through which you can access the internet and email. Course work (case studies and essays) must be wordprocessed.

Warwick There are modern facilities at the medical school and no shortage of computer rooms and clusters around the campus.

Clinical skills
Clinical skills at Leicester begin during the first year of study. This initially takes the form of interviewing "simulated patients" as well as practising physical examination skills on volunteers. This progresses in the second year to clinical placements one morning per week in one of the Leicester hospitals, where the skills learnt in the first year are revised and put into practice.

Welfare

Student support

Leicester The faculty staff at the MSB are very approachable and supportive, and some individual tutors are particularly accessible to discuss problems, etc. Each hospital has a student facilitator to deal with queries and problems. There is always a member of staff available (24 hours) if there are any major problems or emergencies, and also a counselling service at Student Health. Leicester University has a counselling service, and some welfare services are available from the Students' Union. Most areas of the medical school and university have standard disabled access facilities, such as ramps and lifts.

Warwick Students can access the main university counselling and welfare services, as well as those available through the Students' Union. A personal tutor scheme operates in the school and interyear relations are good, so there is always someone you can ask advice from about the course.

Accommodation

Leicester University accommodation is available throughout the degree, and some medical students stay in Putney Road Houses beyond the first year. In the first year it is popular – and advisable – to live in catered halls, as there are loads of activities and great end-of-term balls and parties. Stamford has one of the best summer balls in the country. Privately rented accommodation is inexpensive but variable in quality. It is best to shop around in advance for a good deal. A Union-run accommodation office can help you find places.

Warwick Accommodation in university halls is not guaranteed for one year. However, prospective first-year students are accommodated in nearby university flats in Earlsdon, Canley, and Coventry. Non-medics living out in private accommodation stay mainly in Leamington Spa or one of the areas of Coventry adjacent to the university (Earlsdon, Canley), a bus or car ride away from the campus.

Placements

Leicester Phase I is based on the university campus in the MSB, and Phase II is based in the CSB/Robert Kilpatrick Building at the Leicester Royal Infirmary (LRI). The LRI is only a 10-minute walk from the MSB, and everything is in reasonable proximity. Teaching also takes place at the General and Glenfield Hospitals, which are a short bus ride or, for the energetic, a cycle ride away. The medical school is currently undergoing a £400m investment programme in which a new medical sciences building is planned to be built at the Leicester General Hospital site. Leicester has three teaching hospitals: Leicester Royal Infirmary, Leicester General, and the Glenfield Hospital. In addition, district general hospitals are used in Kettering, Coventry, Nuneaton, Boston, Lincoln, and Peterborough, and free accommodation is provided. GP attachments are in Leicester and the surrounding area, with the furthest away being in Rugby.

Warwick The medical school building is at Gibbet Hill, a quiet part of the campus, a short walk away from the main centre. The brand new buildings are excellent and well equipped (although there are some concerns about a shortage of space already). Students have a nice common room with pigeon holes, some catering facilities, and a balcony. The main teaching hospitals are George Elliot (Nuneaton), Walsgrave, Warwick Hospital, and the Coventry and Warwick Hospital.

Sports and social

City life

Leicester The city centre is about a 45-minute walk from halls, or 10–15 minutes from the university campus. There is a regular bus service between halls, the town centre, and the university during term time. A good range of cinemas, theatres, pubs, clubs, bars, and shops manages to reflect the city's diverse ethnicity. There are plenty of restaurants, and curry lovers in particular have a wide choice of eateries. There are popular clubs in town and late bars to suit all tastes. Many top bands take in Leicester on tour at De Montfort Hall and at De Montfort University. Leicester manages to have all the facilities of a city as well as some of the homeliness and friendliness of a smaller town.

The city is reasonably small, but has recently been redeveloped and has all the shops you could want. If you have a car, the Leicestershire countryside is attractive and makes a pleasant escape from the city. There is football and world-class rugby on the doorstep, and there is a buzz about the place.

Warwick Warwick might have been named Coventry University when it was founded. OK, it may be in Warwickshire, but it is really a part of Coventry. Coventry suffered terribly in the Blitz and much of the centre was unimaginatively rebuilt. One notable exception is the new cathedral, which was built within the remains of the old one. It does, however, have almost everything you might expect of a medium-sized city: theatre, museums, good shopping, restaurants, and travel links. It was the centre of the British car industry and retains Jaguar, Land Rover, and Peugeot plants. Coventry cannot boast the success of Leicester in terms of national sporting prowess, as both its rugby and football teams are no longer Premiership quality. A short journey in any direction can get you into pretty countryside, and places to visit in Warwickshire include Kenilworth Castle, Warwick and Warwick Castle, and Stratford-upon-Avon.

Students at Warwick can take advantage of a wide range of facilities on campus. A large Students' Union provides a wide range of entertainment: bands, balls, and student theatre are all regular events. A large and busy Arts Centre hosts many touring theatre and dance companies, as well as music of all types. Banks, shops, and a post office are all on the doorstep.

Uni life

Leicester At the Students' Union there are club nights every Wednesday, Thursday, Friday, and some Saturdays. Private parties take place at the start of the week. The bar is open all day every weekday, and on Saturday and Sunday nights. Food can be bought during the day. The MedSoc holds parties every term, as well as the Christmas and annual dinners. There are a large variety of university societies to choose from: some are a bit mad, but if you want to join a society you will be spoilt for choice.

Warwick In spite of its relative youth, Warwick has a busy MedSoc which runs regular events for medics. The inaugural student-run freshers' week was a success, with pub crawls, a toga party, and a bowling night being hits with the new students.

Sports life

Leicester There is a wide range of medic sporting teams to choose from, and there have been vast improvements in recent years. Thanks to the enthusiasm of recent MedSoc committees, sponsorship for these teams is now in place. There are sports fields, two sports halls, two gyms, where there are circuits and aerobic classes, and an athletics track. There are plenty of swimming pools in town, or one near the university halls in Oadby.

Warwick There are many sports facilities at Warwick, including an athletics track, swimming pool, playing fields, and sports centre. All the main sports are catered for, as well as many less popular ones.

Great things about Leicester

- Friendly: students are welcoming.
- Phase I faculty staff are very friendly and approachable. They offer a wide range of help, from support with work to trying to help stressed or upset students.
- There are wide-ranging activities available for all organised by MedSoc, the Union, and other societies.
- Great improvement in Leicester's nightlife in recent years, with many new bars, clubs, and restaurants for varying tastes.
- Clinical teaching is done in pairs.

Bad things about Leicester

- Location of placements can present you with travel problems.
- Lack of temperature control in lecture theatres.
- Phase II students are spread about the region.
- Not near the sea. In fact, Leicester is about as far from it as you can be.
- Pink ID badges.

Great things about Warwick

- Brand new building with a state-of-the-art lecture theatre.
- Great Arts Centre on campus.
- Significant clinical content from early on in the course, and clinical application of what is learnt is constantly emphasised.
- State-of-the-art video equipment beams teaching to us from anywhere in the world – well, mainly from Leicester.
- There is some excitement about being part of a new way of doing things.

Bad things about Warwick

- Travel to Leicester for part of the course is time consuming.
- Some of the organisation and timetabling has not been sympathetic to students.

- At the end of a long day it is often a tiring journey home if you live off campus.
- Car parking during the day on campus is expensive, and you sometimes feel as if Warwick University exists purely to make money.
- Some of the student accommodation areas are quite a distance from Phase II DGHs.

Additional application information

Average A-level requirements	AAB (chemistry and biology)
Average Scottish Higher requirements	AAB (chemistry and biology). Must offer CSYS
Make-up of interview panel	Academic/Consultant and final-year medical student
Months in which interviews are held	November–March
Proportion of overseas students	7%
Proportion of mature students	10% (not including graduate school)
Faculty's view of students taking a gap year	Encouraged
Proportion of students taking intercalated degrees	5–10% (n/a for graduate school)
Possibility of direct entrance to clinical phase	Unlikely

	Leicester	Warwick (graduate)
Fees for graduates	£1100	£1100 year 1 only
Fees for overseas students	£9660 preclinical	£18 285 clinical
Assistance for elective funding	Bursary scheme and £250 loan	-
Assistance for travel to attachments	None	None
Access and hardship funds	Available	Available
Weekly rent	Halls £50–£100 Private £40–£45	Halls £45–£55 Private £45
Pint of lager	Union bar £1–£1.50 City centre pub £1.80	Union bar £1.20 City centre pub £1.70
Cinema	£3.50 (with NUS card)	£2.80 (with NUS card)
Nightclub	Free–£5	Free–£10

Further information

Dr Kevin West
Maurice Shock Medical Sciences Building
Leicester University
University Road
Leicester LE1 7RH
Tel: 0116 252 2969/2985
Fax: 0116 252 3013
Email: med-admis@le.ac.uk
Web: http://www.lwms.ac.uk

Liverpool

Key facts	Liverpool
Course length	5 years
Total number of medical undergraduates	1200
Applicants in 2002	1516
Interviews given in 2002	75%
Places available in 2002	268
Places available in 2003	308
Entrance requirements	AAB
Mandatory subjects	Chemistry and biology at A or AS
Male:female ratio	36:64
Premed course	No
Fast-track course	Yes

In 1996 Liverpool Medical School introduced a brand new curriculum, in accordance with GMC guidelines. So far it is proving to be a success. August 2001 saw the first PBL (problem-based learning) students to qualify at Liverpool start on wards as PRHOs. Liverpool Medical School is growing in size, with over 1200 undergraduates, but a strong Medical Students' Society ensures there's always a friendly face around. All this, together with one of the most vibrant cities in the UK, makes for five years you are guaranteed not to forget!

Education

Since the introduction of the new PBL course, subjects are no longer taught in lecture theatres day in, day out: instead, different areas of medicine are presented to students as problems. Students discuss the issues and formulate learning objectives in small groups with tutor guidance. They then go away and research the information for themselves. From the beginning of the second year an increasing proportion of time is spent on hospital and community attachments. Studies follow the human lifecycle, from conception and birth through adulthood and into old age.

Teaching

The new course contains little in the way of formal teaching. The few plenaries (lectures) that are given are designed to provide an overview only of each problem. It is then up to the student to find out further details from the other resources available. Alongside library work, students have formal training in clinical and communication skills. Anatomy is demonstrated using models and prosections in a recently refurbished and improved Human Anatomy Resource Centre. IT (information technology) has an ever-increasing role, with various computer-based learning packages available.

Assessment

Assessment is continuous, designed so that everything you learn (including practical skills acquired) will be recognised and recorded. Formal exams occur in the first, third, and fourth years. There are no exams in the final year! The final year is spent in five, eight-week rotations consisting of two options plus general practice, emergency medicine, and ward shadowing designed to prepare students for the realities of the house job.

Intercalated degrees

It is possible to study for an intercalated degree at the end of the fourth year. Subjects available include anatomy, biochemistry, cell biology, pharmacology, physiology, psychology, and healthcare ethics. Students at Liverpool can study at BSc, BA or Master's level, depending on the degree course taken. Some students study for an intercalated degree at another university and then return to complete the medical course at Liverpool. Limited funding is available to some students wishing to study for an intercalated year.

Special study modules and electives

Elective studies/SSMs, each lasting four weeks, are spread through the first four years of the course. Topics from any specialty can be chosen, and an essay must be completed for each module. An addition to the course are the two SAMPs – selective in advanced medical practice. These are eight-week placements taken as part of the final year, spent in a specialty chosen by the student.

Added opportunities

Two exchange schemes – Socrates and Erasmus – allow students to study at a participating European medical school for a period of 16 weeks during the final year. Current exchanges are set up with schools in France, Germany, Holland, and Sweden. The scheme has recently been expanded to include Eastern European countries.

Facilities

Library A short-loan system operates for the books most in demand. The library is open until 9.30 pm most weekdays. Opening hours are more restricted at weekends and outside the main university terms, which differ from the medical school terms. All hospitals have their own libraries, and borrowing arrangements for students vary.

Computers   The university and hospitals have 24-hour computer facilities available for students, with free use of email and the internet.

Clinical skills   One of the real highlights of the new course has been the introduction of the clinical skills laboratory, where students are able to master a whole range of practical doctoring skills, from taking blood and suturing wounds to giving advanced CPR. There are weekly classes in the first year, with a clinical skills exam at the end. Most students agree it is the best part of the week.

Welfare

Student support

Students generally mix well and there are good relations within and between year groups. There is a long-standing mentoring system set up by the LMSS (Liverpool Medical Students Society), so that each first-year student is paired with a second- or third-year. In recent years Liverpool has enjoyed a very constructive and student-friendly atmosphere within the faculty. In addition to facilities provided by LMSS, the Students' Union has the standard welfare and counselling services.

Accommodation

Most people only live in university accommodation for their first year. This is a good opportunity to meet other students from outside the medical school, but university accommodation is more expensive than renting privately. There is a wide variation in the standard of private accommodation, but there is plenty of choice. The university has no input into regulating the private sector, but the accommodation office can offer advice.

Placements

Liverpool University was the original redbrick university. The campus dominates a large area adjacent to the city centre and between the two cathedrals. The University Hospital is right next to the university campus, and the medical school is well placed near to all the main university and hospital departments.

The medical school is part of a large teaching hospital, the Royal Liverpool University Hospital. Also within the city centre is the Liverpool Women's Hospital, which has 200+ beds. Liverpool has its share of regional specialist centres, including Broadgreen Cardiothoracic Centre, and Alder Hey Children's Hospital in the suburbs. University Hospital Aintree is the other main teaching hospital used by second- and third-year students and is located about six miles from the university.

In the first year all teaching is done in the university. From the second year onwards, more time is spent on placements. For example, on a typical two-week module in the second year, one day is spent in a local GP practice and two days are spent either in a relevant community attachment or at one of the hospitals. Placements are mainly within or near to Liverpool (Wirral, Southport, Warrington, Halton, etc.), but some are further away, such as Rhyl (North Wales) and Chester. In the final year placements can be as far away as Llandudno in North Wales, and Barrow-in-Furness in the Lake District.

Sports and social

City life

Liverpool offers an excellent welcome to students. It is a proud yet warm city, with its world-famous accent, sense of humour, two cathedrals, football teams, and maritime history. It was once the biggest port in the British Empire. Having fallen on hard times in the 1970s and 1980s, Liverpool is now very much on the up! Many students, from all courses, stay in the area after graduation. The medical school and the student residential areas are well placed for all the attractions, and are adjacent to the many parks within the city. Like many other cities there is crime about, but a commonsense approach will ensure that the good times aren't spoilt. Police statistics show that Liverpool is, in fact, one of the safest cities in the UK.

Liverpool has an excellent social side – every food taste catered for, excellent pubs, several cinemas, sports complexes, and nightclubs of all hues, from 70s clubs upwards. It is also the home of two great football teams (Liverpool and Tranmere Rovers), and one other (Everton); the world's most famous horse race, the Grand National at Aintree (oh, have we mentioned The Beatles yet?). The city is only a short distance from Manchester, North Wales, Chester, and the Lake District.

Uni life

LMSS has weekly meetings with guest speakers. There are regular balls, dinners, and social parties, as well as the medics' own orchestra, choir, sports teams, play, and Christmas revue. The university also offers a wide range of different societies. LMSS has its own website at http://www.LMSS.org. There is also a very active and expanding branch of MedSIN.

Sports life

The Medical Society has football, rugby, hockey, netball, basketball, squash, badminton, and cricket teams. Recent additions to the sports teams include Chinese martial arts and a celebrated tiddlywinks team! The university has all these and more! There are plenty of facilities.

Great things about Liverpool

- The PBL course is self-directed and self-motivated, and allows you to adapt your learning to your pace.
- Students have a real say in the course at Liverpool, and course organisers are receptive to their suggestions.
- The course prepares students to work effectively as PRHOs through early patient contact and clinical skills training.

- During the early years, the self-directed nature of the course allows students to make time to pursue other interests – in effect, the course is on flexitime.
- The LMSS provides a strong backbone to all activities in Liverpool Medical School, from academic issues to social and welfare issues.

Bad things about Liverpool

- The necessary approach to course work at Liverpool can be very different from A-level studies: PBL is not for people who want to be spoon-fed in lectures.
- Hospital placements can be some distance from Liverpool, and travelling by public transport can be time consuming and expensive.
- The constant evaluation form filling can become tiresome.
- University facilities are available during university term dates. Outside these "normal term times", facilities such as the library are operated on restricted "vacation hours".
- The social life within the medical school can be so good that sometimes it is difficult to get to know students from other courses!

Additional application information

Average A-level requirements	• Two science subjects at A-level (grades AB) must be offered. Biology and chemistry must be taken at AS-level if not A-level. Additionally another A-level subject at grade A (or equivalent)
Average Scottish Higher requirements	• AAABB – including chemistry, biology, maths, physics, English. Two Advanced Highers, including chemistry
Make-up of interview panel	• Two senior clinical and academic staff
Months in which interviews are held	• November–March
Proportion of overseas students	• 6%
Proportion of mature students	• 20%
Faculty's view of students taking a gap year	• Encouraged as long as the year has broad educational benefit
Proportion of students taking intercalated degrees	• 10%
Possibility of direct entrance to clinical phase	• No
Fees for graduates	• £1100
Fees for overseas students	• £15 800 pa
Assistance for elective funding	• c. £12 000 pa to be divided on merit between student applicants
Assistance for travel to attachments	• Some is being phased in for final-year students at distant GP placements
Access and hardship funds	• Any full-time UK student can apply for hardship awards but there are no guaranteed funds
Weekly rent	• Halls £51–£83 Private £37–£60
Pint of lager	• Union bar £1 + City centre pub £1–£3
Cinema	• £3+
Nightclub	• Free–£12

Further information

Admissions Administrator
Faculty of Medicine
1st floor Duncan Building
Daulby Street
Liverpool L69 3GA
Tel: 0151 706 4266
Fax: 0151 706 5667
Email: mbchb@liv.ac.uk
Web: http://www.liv.ac.uk

Manchester, Keele and Preston

Key facts	Manchester	Keele
Course length	5 years	5 years
Total number of medical undergraduates	c. 1500	155
Applicants in 2002	1920	N/A
Interviews given in 2002	823	N/A
Places available in 2002	340	N/A
Places available in 2003	340	Year 1:55, Year 3:50
Entrance requirements	AAB	AAB
Mandatory subjects	Chemistry	Chemistry
Male:female ratio	42:58	N/A
Premed course	Yes	No
Fast-track course	No	No

Manchester

Manchester is home to three universities: the University of Manchester, the Manchester Metropolitan University (MMU), and the University of Manchester Institute of Science and Technology (UMIST). As a result, it boasts a student population of over 50 000. The medical school is part of the University of Manchester and is the second largest in the UK. Medicine has been on the curriculum here since the early 19th century.

The medical campus is situated on Oxford Road, right in the heart of a busy cosmopolitan city, which many now see as the London of the North. In 1994 Manchester was the first UK school to introduce a new systems-based problem-based learning curriculum, following the publication of the GMC document *Tomorrow's Doctors*, and so has over eight years' experience in problem-based learning. Although a preclinical/clinical divide exists, the basic sciences are studied within a clinical framework of patient cases, which are used to direct learning each week.

Manchester is unique in that students are joined in the third year by an intake of students from St Andrew's. In addition, students may choose to undertake part or all of their training at the new teaching centre of Keele.

Preston, a base hospital of the Lancashire Teaching Hospital NHS Trust, will welcome its first group of year 3 students in September 2003. This new base hospital is a permanent addition to the Manchester Medical Schools and will provide additional medical education posts in the north west.

Education

The course is five years long, with two preclinical years followed by three clinical ones. The preclinical course is structured around weekly cases that are studied through a mixture of group discussion, practical anatomy and pathology laboratories, computer skills sessions, lecture theatre events, and personal study. The course is organised into four semesters, so that cases relate to the four themes of nutrition and metabolism, cardiorespiratory, abilities and disabilities, and lifecycle. Years 3 and 4 continue the case-based approach in a clinical setting, and the four themes are repeated. Four days per week are spent in one of the five teaching hospitals, and one day per week in general practice surgery. The fifth year works on a four-block rotation system, whereby an equal number of students will be on an elective, at a teaching hospital, a district general hospital, or in the community at any one time. Because of the high attendance demands on final-year students, free hospital accommodation is provided during attachments, which allows students to shadow house officers and gain practical experience to prepare them for their preregistration house jobs.

Teaching

First- and second-year teaching focuses on a weekly case study with supplementary group discussions, lectures, and practical sessions, including microscopy, anatomy, group tutorials, anatomy sessions using cadavers, basic clinical skills, and computational skills. Students work in groups to create weekly learning objectives, which are fulfilled in their own time with the aid of the above resources.

Years 3, 4, and 5 continue to base teaching around a case setting, but students now fulfil learning objectives within a clinical setting. Whereas in the first year the study objectives in the case of the man with lung cancer would involve learning about the pathology of lung cancers from a textbook and pathology specimens, in clinical years students would have the opportunity to attend chest clinics and talk to and examine people with the actual disease. In the clinical years, students also receive bedside teaching. In years 3 and 4 there is a maximum of 12 students per firm. Unfortunately, it is not uncommon for sessions to be cancelled, or for sessions to be rescheduled owing to patient commitments of the medical staff.

Assessment

In years 1 and 2 there are exams at the end of each of the four semesters. They comprise MCQs, two papers on clinical case studies, an exam requiring the interpretation of scientific prose into lay language, an OSSE (objective structured skills examination) and, unusually, a computer skills exam.

At the end of each semester groups are assessed and marked for communication skills and teamwork. For those studying the "European option" there are weekly lessons with homework and exams.

Assessment in years 3 and 4 is twice a year and consists of a true/false paper and an OSCE. The OSCE sees students rotate through up to 15 five-minute stations, where they are presented with various tasks and challenges appropriate to the area they are being assessed upon. For example, students may be asked to interpret laboratory results, examine patients, or deal with ethically challenging situations. In the final year, students take one set of exams in May comprising an OSCE, a patient management paper (PMP) and a final true/false paper.

Intercalated degrees

Intercalated BSc courses are offered at the end of the second, third, or fourth years. There is a wide range of basic bioscience subjects available to study, as well as more unusual subjects such as healthcare ethics and law, and history of medicine, which have proved extremely popular over recent years. Traditionally, students wishing to intercalate would have been expected to have an above average academic record, but faculty seem to be widening access to any student wishing to intercalate. Some funding is available, and is allocated according to academic merit. Some scholarships are also available from businesses, depending on the subject studied.

Special study modules and electives

In years 1 and 2 there is one four-week special study module (SSM) per year, whereas in years 3 and 4 there are two per year. These modules can be on practically anything, and there is talk of allowing students to do one SSM in a topic unrelated to medicine to encourage the pursuit of other hobbies and interests. Another point to note is that in the clinical years one of the SSMs must be in a DGH (district general hospital) and one in the community.

Many students do SSMs at Preston; the Families and Children module has been run at Preston for several years now. Both Chorley and South Ribble DGH have a good record in providing year 5 placements in hospital and community for the Preston course.

In the final year there is an elective period, where students are encouraged to go abroad to appreciate medical education in a foreign healthcare setting. The elective officially lasts eight weeks, but students often piggyback their time on to an adjacent holiday such as Christmas to increase their time away. Students cover costs for electives, so a great deal of organisation and planning is often needed. In addition, a report must be submitted upon returning to Manchester.

Added opportunities

Eligible Manchester students are also offered the chance to pursue the "European option". Students who successfully complete this element of the course are awarded a degree which recognises their medical training in the context of a foreign language and healthcare system. Students with good grades in A-level languages can choose to study either French or German in addition to the medicine course. Medical vocabulary is taught from year 1, and four months of year 5 are spent at the partner universities of Rennes (France), Saarland (Germany), and Lausanne (Switzerland). The faculty has established good working relationships with these three faculties over a number of years and knows that students receive experience equivalent to that in Manchester.

Uniquely to Manchester, at the end of the fourth year students undertake a 12-week research project. Students are allocated a supervisor and have the opportunity to pursue a topic that particularly interests them. This period provides an excellent introduction to medical research, and allows students to get to grips with medical statistics. Some students even go on to have their work published.

Students may also interrupt the course to complete a PhD.

Facilities

Library   The Medical Faculty library is well equipped with the basic textbooks, but demand is high and it is often busy. It is open 9 am–8 pm during term time, weekdays only. The John Rylands University Library across the road stocks most of the major journals. This library is open from 9 am to 9.30 pm weekdays, and 9 am–6 pm and 1 pm–6 pm on Saturday and Sunday, respectively. The opening hours in holiday times are shorter. Hospital libraries vary in size and standard.

Computers   There are excellent computer facilities in the medical school and John Rylands Library, with internet access and email for all. A number of computer-assisted learning programs are available, and computer laboratories in the medical school are open from 9 am to 7 pm. Hospitals also have computer and email facilities.

Clinical skills   More and more emphasis is being placed on the use of skills laboratories, and facilities in the clinical years of the course are being improved. There has been a tremendous influx of cash into the skills laboratories over the last two years and there is a variety of mannequins for practising CPR, injections, blood taking, etc., and video resources on clinical skills.

Welfare

Student support

Faculty staff are extremely approachable and student feedback is consistently encouraged. Student representatives sit on all major faculty committees, and student opinions are frequently sought. In particular, three staff–student liaison meetings are held in each academic year, which give ample opportunity for students to raise issues close to their hearts. Good relationships between students and tutors are fostered through tutorials. Students are also allocated a member of staff who acts as a pastoral tutor, and there are both faculty and Students' Union-based counselling services, which are highly regarded.

Accommodation

University accommodation is guaranteed for first-years, and although most students choose to move into the private sector after this, many do stay. Halls may be catered or self-catering, and vary in price and standard. There is a lot of private sector accommodation, ranging in price from £37 to £60 per week. Most accommodation is within walking distance of the university, and a short bus ride from the town centre. The last few years have also seen the rise of a number of large commercial accommodation blocks aimed at students, a number of which offer rooms with en-suite facilities, and even onsite gyms and swimming pools!

Placements

In years 3 and 4, four days per week are spent at the base hospital and one day in the community. However, it is worth noting that, as in most other medical schools, getting to and from placements can be time consuming without a car. In theory, base hospitals (excluding Keele and Preston) are all within 45 minutes of the university by public transport. However, although having a car can be a general advantage in the clinical years, the public transport network is fast and efficient and often beats rush-hour traffic.

Sports and social

City life

With such a huge student population, Manchester offers an endless choice of where to go and what to do. There is a wide variety of pubs, bars, clubs, stores, theatres, and restaurants, each with a different character, theme, or style. The city is truly multicultural and there is a good mix of home, overseas, mature, and postgraduate students, as well as a vibrant gay and lesbian scene. The music scene (post Acid and "Madchester") is on the up, and as well as the local scene, most of the big-name tours include Manchester gigs. However, should all the excitement get too much for you, the Peak District, Pennines, Lake District, and North Wales are not far away for a little peace and tranquillity, along with Liverpool, Leeds, and Sheffield!

Uni life

The Medical Students' Representative Council (MSRC) is the focus of medical school social life. The 12-strong committee is elected each year by students and organises a number of medics' events throughout the year, including the famous pyjama pub crawl and the annual winter ball. There are also year clubs, which organise trips, parties, and one graduation ball for each year. The medics run an orchestra, a dramatics society, which organises an annual pantomime, and a revue. In addition, the medical school magazine *Mediscope* is published three times a year (on paper and the web) and provides a journalistic forum for the medical student population. Along with faculty events, a huge range of clubs and societies are run from Manchester Students' Union, which is opposite the medical school.

Sports life

Being home to the most famous football team in the world is only the start for Manchester, and although tickets for United's games can be a little pricey, Manchester City offers cut-price tickets to students for home games. This is probably a blessing in disguise, as the majority of locals living in the student areas are City fans! There is also a discount price for students at Sale Sharks Rugby Club.

Manchester's sports scene has seen huge benefits from the opening of many facilities built to cater for the 2002 Commonwealth Games, which has left a legacy of world-class sporting facilities. Developments include a campus-located Olympic size hi-tech swimming pool, as well as the creation of the national cycling, squash, and netball centres. The centrepiece of the Commonwealth Games is the 37 000-seat "City of Manchester stadium", which in 2003 will become the new home of Manchester City.

Within the medical school, Manchester has a thriving sporting community. There are medics' rugby, hockey, tennis, netball, rowing, and football teams, which actively encourage participation and socialising. The main university also has countless sports clubs, but medics tend to play for the medics' team if one exists in their sport. A brilliant annual tour also takes place for each medics' sport team.

Keele

The Universities of Manchester and Keele won funding to provide training and education for undergraduate medics from October 2000 onwards, and also to establish the full five-year course at Keele from September 2003. Students who wish to study at Keele have the following options.

- Five-year course at Keele.
- Five-year course with years 1 and 2 at Manchester and the final three years at Keele.
- Six-year course, including a premedical year for students without an appropriate science background at A-level. The premedical year is at Manchester.

An intercalated degree can be incorporated with any of the options. The BSc can be taken at Keele or Manchester. Keele hopes to offer the European option from 2003.

Keele University is offering undergraduate medical education in partnership with Manchester University. Depending on your choice of the study options listed above, you should apply to either Manchester or Keele (K12). Students undertaking the full five-year course at Keele will spend years 1 and 2 based primarily on the Keele campus site in the new purpose-built Health Sciences complex.

Keele is a large attractive campus university with restaurants, social and sports facilities, as well as library and academic buildings. The clinical years at Keele will be spent predominantly at the North Staffordshire NHS Hospital Trust, only three miles away from Keele. This is a very busy hospital offering the full range of clinical services and an excellent place to gain clinical experience. In addition, students are guaranteed accommodation on campus for their first year of study.

The structure of the course and the assessments are the same for both Keele and Manchester students. The first students for Keele and North Staffordshire will arrive in October 2002, having started in Manchester in October 2000. Plans are progressing well to ensure that the additional academic and clinical facilities are in place. New staff will be recruited in the early part of 2002, as well as the responsibilities of existing staff being changed. The local consultants and staff in partner district general hospitals are extremely enthusiastic about the new school and are looking forward to the first group of students arriving.

Preston: Lancashire teaching hospitals

Preston forms part of the Lancashire teaching hospitals and was created in August 2002 by the merger of two well-established hospitals. Royal Preston Hospital has a long history and is now a modern building with good transport access. Chorley and South Ribble DGH was extensively rebuilt and enlarged in 1994. Both hospitals have an excellent record in providing placements for Manchester students.

From September 2003 the Lancashire teaching hospitals will have 30 places per annum for Manchester students; from 2007 this will increase up to 80 places. Students in the first phase will benefit from superior staff–student ratios and access to clinical cases.

There is a modern education unit at the Chorley site and a new education and training unit under construction at Preston to provide state-of-the-art facilities for learning and teaching. Both centres will have excellent library and IT resources in addition to a well-provided clinical skills unit.

Student accommodation will be available within a reasonable distance from the main base hospital at Preston. Access to Manchester is reasonable, journeys are 30–40 minutes by car. Trains are frequent and provide access to central Manchester in 30–40 minutes. Blackpool, Preston and Wigan have an active nightlife and Preston has a large student population linked to the University of Central Lancashire.

For further information Dr Simon Wallis, Director of Medical Education and Hospital Dean, may be contacted on 01257 245 600 or email simon.wallis@LTHTR.nhs.uk

Great things about Manchester

- Enthusiasm for medicine is maintained by a course that emphasises clinical problems from day 1.
- The faculty staff are very approachable and open to change. There are plenty of opportunities to give feedback on both course and staff.
- The social life is excellent. There are loads of events organised by the MSRC (Medical Students' Representative Council) and there is generally lots going on at reasonable prices.
- The sheer size of the multifaculty universities in Manchester, and the 2002 Commonwealth Games, have ensured top-level academic and sporting facilities.
- In the third year a load of new people arrive from St Andrew's, which spices things up a bit!

Bad things about Manchester

- Adjusting to self-directed learning can be difficult for some students who are used to being spoon-fed, although this is becoming the case at all UK schools with new courses.
- Differing interpretations of self-directed learning can often mean students perceive a lack of teaching.
- Some hospital placements are quite a distance away and can be difficult to reach on public transport.
- Manchester does have a higher than average crime rate and insurance premiums are in the more expensive bands.
- It has a habit of raining like hell.

Additional application information

Average A-level requirements	• AAB, including chemistry
Average Scottish Higher requirements	• AAAAB
Make-up of interview panel	• Three consultants and one bioscientist or GP, with a mix of specialties, genders and ethnicities
Months in which interviews are held	• November–April
Proportion of overseas students	• 6–7%
Proportion of mature students	• 10%
Faculty's view of students taking a gap year	• Neutral
Proportion of students taking intercalated degrees	• 20–30 students each year
Possibility of direct entrance to clinical phase	• Low
Fees for graduates	• £1100
Fees for overseas students	• Check with medical school
Assistance for elective funding	• Scholarships and prizes available
Assistance for travel to attachments	• Via Local Education Authority
Access and hardship funds	• Yes, via Dept. of Awards and Exams

	Manchester	Keele
Weekly rent	Halls £47–£77 Private £37–£60	Halls £42.40–£70 all self-catering; private £36–£50 depending on letting period and type of accommodation·
Pint of lager	Union bar £1.50 City centre pub £1.90	Union bar £1 before 10 pm, £1.55 after 10 pm; city centre pub £1.80–£2
Cinema	£2.50 with student ID	Keele Film Society on campus offers weekly programme – tickets £2 Multiscreen Odeon cinema at Festival Park, Hanley – £3.60, Warner Village – £3 (with union card); Stoke Film Theatre (Staffordshire University) tickets £2.50
Nightclub	Free–£12	N/A

Further information

Manchester
Ms L M Harding
Admissions Officer
Faculty of Medicine
Stopford Building
University of Manchester
Oxford Road
Manchester M13 9PT
Tel: 0161 275 2077
Fax: 0161 275 5697
Email: ug.admissions@man.ac.uk
Web: http://www.man.ac.uk

Keele
Admissions and Recruitment Office
School of Medicine
The Covert
Keele University
Staffordshire ST5 5BG
Tel: 01782 583632/583642
Fax: 01782 583903
Email: medicine@keele.ac.uk
Web: http://www.keele.ac.uk

Until 2007 at the earliest, Keele can only consider applications from home and EU students.

Newcastle and UDSC (Durham)

Key facts	Newcastle	Durham
Course length	5 years	5 years
Total number of medical undergraduates	965	140
Applicants in 2002	1326	317
Interviews given in 2002	56%	62%
Places available in 2002	220	70
Places available in 2003	245	95
Entrance requirements	AAB	AAB
Mandatory subjects	Chemistry or biology	Chemistry or biology
Male:female ratio	35:65	45:55
Premed course	Yes	Yes
Fast-track course	Yes	No

Newcastle is a friendly city and the university is very centrally situated. The medical school is five minutes away from the main campus, very near to the halls of residence. As in the rest of the university there is a diversity of students, both national and international, from many different backgrounds. The staff are generally approachable and supportive, and well liked by students. Following extensive building work in 2000/01 the medical school is proud to have a brand new, state-of-the-art 400-seat lecture theatre.

Early patient contact comes from hospital and GP visits in the first two years, and the course has broken down the traditional preclinical/clinical divide. There are opportunities for extended contact with patients by way of the "family" and "patient" studies (see below). The social life, centred on both the university and the city itself, is excellent, with something to appeal to everyone. Newcastle, the northernmost English university city, gives a warm welcome to its students.

The University of Durham has opened a new medical degree course at its Stockton campus (UDSC). Seventy students began Phase I of the Newcastle MBBS programme in September 2001. Students spend the first two years of the course at UDSC before being integrated with the much larger numbers of Newcastle students in years 3–5. The course in Stockton has been developed alongside that in Newcastle. It aims to produce a cohort of students with the same levels of skills and knowledge as those produced via the more traditional route in Newcastle. Although the two courses work to similar terminal objectives, there are some key differences on the UDSC course, which we have highlighted in the profile. The campus is based at Stockton, in an attractive part of town amid a redeveloped riverside. Stockton is a small and friendly place, and although it might not boast all the attractions of a big city it has all the facilities you would expect of a big town.

UDSC has developed strong links with schools and colleges of education in the local area through visits and a programme of targeted promotional open days. Students on the course have qualifications ranging from the usual science A-levels to a wide range of first and second degrees, as well as professional qualifications from the worlds of law, nursing, physiology, and radiography.

Students at Newcastle quickly develop an affection for this vibrant, rapidly developing city, and the large student presence makes for an excellent social life. Although Stockton is a fairly small town, nearby Middlesbrough offers a wide range of evening entertainment.

Education

The courses at Newcastle and UDSC are divided into two major phases based on the traditional preclinical/clinical model. Each is subdivided into two stages. In years 1 and 2 the course is case led and systems based, becoming more clinically relevant as you progress through. The university has no intention of moving to a solely problem-based learning model, but Phase I of the course does include case-based work. The preclinical/clinical divide is reducing, and there are several opportunities for early patient contact in the form of project work, hospital and GP visits, and patient presentations. Practical skills, such as taking blood, are taught from term 1 of the first year. The "family" project links a student with a local mother-to-be and encourages the student to share as much as possible in the experience of pregnancy through the eyes of the woman and her family.

The main distinguishing feature of the course at Stockton is the 30 hours per semester spent in placements selected from a variety of local voluntary and community groups. Student reports and reflections from these placements count towards assessment in year 2.

Teaching

Teaching is in two phases: Phase I is conducted over two sites, Newcastle and Stockton, and in Phase II all students combine to form one cohort and are allocated into one of four base units around the region. These are

- **Teesside** (Cleveland and Middlesbrough)
- **Wear** (hospitals south of the Tyne down to Durham)
- **Tyne** (central Newcastle hospitals and the Queen Elizabeth Hospital in Gateshead), and
- **Northumbria** (Northumberland, Hexham, and Carlisle).

There is a degree of choice over which base unit you are allocated to, and most students end up with their first or second choice. Certain extenuating circumstances may guarantee a particular base unit.

In Phase I (two years, consists of stages 1 and 2) approximately 40% of study time is spent in lectures, small group seminars, and practical sessions. Anatomy classes use prosected specimens. Following a GMC visit in 1998 and a curriculum review, timetabled hours have decreased in the first two years, leaving students more "white" time. Wednesday afternoons are free for sport across the university.

Phase II (three years, consisting of stages 3 and 4) sees the emphasis shift significantly to clinical experience, and teaching takes place further afield in the region. There is an introductory "clinical skills" course, lasting 16 weeks, which introduces students systematically and thoroughly to clinical history taking and examination, and is one of the best received parts of the course by students. After this, students embark on a series of essential junior rotations which takes them through to the first part of final examinations in November of year 4.

Stage 4 of Phase II begins in January of the fourth year with 21 weeks of student-selected special study modules (SSMs). The nine-week elective period (plus two weeks' holiday) follows. Final year consists of essential senior rotations in the major clinical specialties. Placements can be throughout the north – from Whitehaven in the west to North Shields in the east, Bishop Auckland in the south to Ashington in the north. Final-year students spend five days a week in hospital and are expected to become part of the team to which they are attached, including being around during some evenings. The emphasis is on taking responsibility for one's own self-directed learning, and therefore time is often left deliberately unstructured.

Assessment

Phase I exams consist of a multiple-choice paper, a data interpretation paper, and a clinical-based objective structured clinical exam (OSCE). In Phase I exams are at the end of each semester, and about six weeks into the first year there is a short MCQ which gives students a chance to see how they're doing. There are also several in-course assessments. Phase II exams (early in year 4) consist of data/problem-solving papers, MCQs, and an OSCE. In-course assessment is by way of in-course marks for the junior rotations and a 5000-word literature review. Final exams at the end of the fifth year consist of data interpretation, an OSCE, and a "long case".

Intercalated degrees

Students who do very well on the course are encouraged to intercalate, after either the second or the fourth year, and study for the additional degree of BMedSci. Research projects are wide ranging, from clinical to laboratory-based work, and topics in the social sciences. About 10% of the students at Newcastle intercalate. UDSC students will intercalate after joining Phase II.

Special study modules and electives

An SSM has been introduced to Phase I. Stage 4 (year 4 term 2, after stage 3 exams) begins with three student-selected modules lasting seven weeks each, where hospital-, community-, and investigative-based topics are studied in depth. This is followed by an 11-week elective period, usually spent abroad.

Facilities

Library   The Newcastle Medical Library is situated within the medical school and is open until 10 pm during the week, but daytime only at weekends. It is well stocked with books and videos, but does get busy at exam time. Students may also use the university library, which is also close to the medical school (five minutes' walk). There are facilities at Stockton, but it will take time to build up the medical information resources.

Computers   These tend to be very good, and much information is passed on to students via email. Computer courses are held as part of the course, specifically in wordprocessing and the use of email/internet to search databases. There are 115 general-access PCs in Newcastle Medical School, with an additional 10 stations for email only. Opening hours are the same as the library. If these are busy, there are numerous quieter clusters throughout the university available for use. There are computer facilities at Stockton.

Clinical skills   Clinical skills are emphasised very early in the course and form an integral part of the exams. The clinical skills laboratory at Newcastle is available for private revision sessions as well as for timetabled teaching sessions.

Welfare

Student support

All students are assigned a personal tutor for pastoral support, and faculty staff are friendly and approachable. The university and Students' Union have a number of welfare officers and counselling services, including Nightline. All fresher medics join a peer family (often with five generations!) to help get themselves orientated. Those at UDSC have families in Newcastle as well, to encourage integration of the courses.

Accommodation

Newcastle freshers' accommodation is guaranteed in halls or self-catering flats, although not all are centrally located. The housing office offers help and advice to students renting in the private sector, as most do from year 2. Popular student areas for renting are Jesmond, Heaton, and Fenham. UDSC offers an excellent standard of reasonably priced student accommodation, both on campus (en-suite) and off.

Placements

The Newcastle campus is situated very close to the city centre and includes the Royal Victoria Infirmary (adjoining the medical school). There is ample opportunity to mix with non-medical students, and at the same time the facilities within the medical school itself are good (refectories, gym, etc.). UDSC is on the Stockton campus, and the smaller numbers lead to good opportunities for integration with both other UDSC students and those from the other Durham colleges. The buildings at Stockton are all very new and are on a stretch of the bank of the Tees which has seen a lot of investment and redevelopment. During Phase II attachments may be much further afield at base units. There is usually good accommodation provided. Travel expenses are currently partially reimbursed, although this is under review.

All but the Teesside base unit are fairly easily accessible, but students do not receive any expenses for their travel costs from Newcastle to their base unit, only to the various hospitals from within the base unit. Those students in the Teesside unit may well be expected to reside there for the year. The disadvantages of considerable commuting distances are often outweighed by the advantage that the smaller district general hospitals further afield usually have fewer students than the central teaching hospitals, and therefore overall enthusiasm for students and teaching facilities are generally excellent.

Sports and social

City life

Newcastle is a very lively city located within easy reach of the hills of Northumberland and the northeast coast of England. Recently voted eighth best party town in the world, there is no shortage of bars and pubs, and an ever-increasing club scene. The medical school has good access to the city centre shops, theatre, cinema, museums, art galleries, and music venues. More shops are to be found at the Metrocentre, just across the River Tyne in Gateshead. The locals are generally very friendly and eager for everyone to have a good time. Crime does not seem to be a major problem in most areas, but bikes do get stolen from time to time.

Stockton is nestled between the bustle of Middlesbrough and Durham, with easy access to both, and to other cities in the north east. In Middlesbrough pubs and clubs abound and you can always take a bus into Durham or Newcastle. There is a shopping complex with a multiplex cinema just minutes from the campus.

Uni life

Students at Newcastle quickly develop an affection for this vibrant, rapidly developing city, and the large student presence makes for an excellent social life. Aalthough Stockton is a fairly small town, nearby Middlesbrough offers a wide range of evening entertainment. MedSoc events take place in Newcastle every Friday evening, and usually consist of a guest speaker or show followed by a free bar; there are also karaoke nights, blind date, man-o-man. The annual MedSoc–DentSoc challenge is a regular favourite. The third-years stage a medics' revue in May, and there are numerous medics' balls and dinners throughout the year. A wide range of other societies are available through the Union. As well as the usual array of pubs, bars, and clubs to suit all tastes in the city centre, a string of new restaurants and bars have recently sprung up in the popular student residential area of Jesmond. At Stockton a MedSoc was established in the first semester, and both it and the BMA's intraschool committee are active.

Sports life

Medics' rugby, netball, and hockey teams compete in leagues, and there are also football, volleyball, cricket, squash, and other sports clubs for medics, and innumerable other university-run clubs. The medical school in Newcastle has its own gym (£7 per year), and the university sports facilities are good and close by (£45 per year). For the enthusiastic supporter there is Newcastle United Football Club, as well as rugby, basketball, and many more professional sports teams.

Great things about Newcastle

- Friendly locals in a vibrant, rapidly developing city where the atmosphere is never impersonal.
- Cost of living is relatively low.
- If you need a break from city life, it's easy to escape to the country or the coast.
- New pubs, clubs, and restaurants spring up all the time, and the exciting new development on the quayside is putting Newcastle and Gateshead firmly in the running for the European Capital of Culture 2008.
- Free beer at MedSoc (for life!).

Bad things about Newcastle

- There is some trepidation about how the new developments with UDSC and the increase in student numbers might affect course organisation and the student body.
- Travelling around the region can be time consuming without a car and costly with one.
- The exam system has been changed several times and this has had an unsettling effect, although the current system has been up and running for three years now.
- The tutor system doesn't work for everyone (efforts are being made to improve the scheme).
- Some consultants mutter bitter words to the effect of "Of course, the students at Newcastle don't know any anatomy these days ..." You'll get sick of hearing it!

Great things about UDSC

- Brand new state-of-the-art facilities, with committed staff.
- Small (165 total medical students from 2002).
- Easy access to Middlesbrough, Durham, and Newcastle.
- Access to both of Durham and Newcastle University facilities, e.g. libraries.
- Integrated, person-centred, socially aware focus of study.

Bad things about UDSC

- The library is still being developed.
- There are very few past examination papers to look at.
- Stockton is a small town.
- Late transport from Durham/Newcastle can be a problem.
- UDSC's reputation has still to be established.

Additional application information

	Newcastle	Durham
Average A-level requirements	• AAB, must include chemistry and/or biology. The school also requires at least AAAAB at GCSE, including maths, science, and English language	
Average Scottish Higher requirements	• AAAAB including English and maths. Also four at grade 1 and a grade 2, including chemistry and biology	
Make-up of interview panel	• Two members from a pool of academic and clinical staff and lay members	
Months in which interviews are held	• Mid-November to mid-February	
Proportion of overseas students	6%	0%
Proportion of mature students	8%	28.5%
Faculty's view of students taking a gap year	• Not a problem as long as applicant has structured plans for the year	
Proportion of students taking intercalated degrees	10% (variable)	Not applicable
Possibility of direct entrance to clinical phase	• Yes, for certain groups of graduates	Not applicable
Fees for graduates	• £1100 pa	£1100 pa
Fees for overseas students	• Phase I £9465 pa Phase II £17 525 pa	Not applicable
Assistance for elective funding	• No	Not applicable
Assistance for travel to attachments	• Yes	Not applicable
Access and hardship funds	• Yes	Yes
Weekly rent	• Halls £64 Private £25–£60	Halls £59.50 Private £28
Pint of lager	• Union bar £1.20 City centre pub £1.50	Union bar £1.20 City centre pub £1.50
Cinema	• £3.00 (with NUS card)	£2.80 (with NUS card)
Nightclub	• Free–£8	50p–£15

Further information

The Medical School
University of Newcastle
Framlington Place
Newcastle Upon Tyne NE2 4HH
Tel: 0191 222 7034
Fax: 0191 222 6139
Email: admission-enquiries@ncl.ac.uk
Web: http://www.ncl.ac.uk, http://medical.faculty.ncl.ac.uk/undergrad/medicine

Nottingham

Key facts	Undergraduate	Graduate entry
Course length	5 years	4 years
Total number of medical students	Approx. 1200	
Applicants in 2002	Over 2000	–
Interviews given in 2002	20%	–
Places available in 2002	245	–
Places available in 2003	245	90
Entrance requirements	AAB in any order	2:2 degree or better
Mandatory subjects	Chemistry and biology	Any degree discipline plus GAMSAT exam
Male:female ratio	35:65	–
Premed course	No	No
Fast-track course	No	Yes

Nottingham is a campus university with a community atmosphere in a vibrant city. Medics and non-medics mix in the first year in superb halls of residence on a beautiful campus built around a lake. There is plentiful off-campus accommodation, mostly located in the Lenton area between the campus and the city. This area is very student orientated, so that many of your friends will live within walking distance of your home(s) throughout the course. The cost of living compares favourably with other university towns, and the city is very multicultural. The medical school is a part of the massive Queen's Medical Centre (QMC) hospital at the city end of the university campus. The course is systems based, with emphasis on the early introduction of clinical skills. Outside placements are accessible and the quality of teaching is high. All students do a BMedSci degree within the five-year course, and there are growing opportunities to study abroad. Clinical attachments are assessed individually and within themselves. The elective follows finals and this is a great idea, allowing less worry and more knowledge. Most graduates choose to find PRHO jobs through the matching scheme and stay in the Nottingham area.

Education

Nottingham offers a blend between traditional and modern-style courses. Throughout the five years the subjects are split into four themes (cell, body, community, and communication/social – learn this for the interview!). The first two years are integrated clinically, with systems-based teaching arranged in four semesters. One morning every fortnight is spent seeing patients, either in general practice or in hospital; clinical skills are taught and examined in both years. Year 3 is split into two halves: the first involves a research project leading to a BMedSci degree for everybody; the second marks the beginning of full-time clinical study, with general medical and surgical attachments after a brief introductory course. The final two years are spent on clinical attachments in a variety of specialties before returning to general medicine and surgery. Throughout the course there is a large but appropriate emphasis on personal and professional development; this includes communication skills, ethics, and career advice.

Teaching

Lectures form the basis of most first- and second-year courses and the main lecture theatres were renovated earlier this year, with new comfy seats. Lectures are supplemented with a limited number of tutorials (about 10 students) and seminars (about 25 students). Anatomy is taught by group dissection (10 students) and clinical problem solving in the newly renovated dissection laboratories. Practical classes are taught in large telelinked laboratories.

Assessment

The course is examined by continual assessment instead of a single final exam after the five years. Depending on your outlook, this either reduces or spreads the inevitable stress. For the first two years exams take place in January and June, often using MCQs, i.e. negatively marked true and false questions (these can be more challenging than they sound). Students are encouraged to give feedback, which sometimes results in improvements. The BMedSci is assessed mainly from a 10 000–15 000-word research-based project. In the clinical years logbook assessment and practical exams follow each attachment, with MCQ exams twice a year. In the fifth year the finals are clinically orientated, involving medicine, surgery, orthopaedics, and clinical laboratory sciences; this year it has been redesigned to allow several practice attempts at finals before the real exam.

Intercalated degrees

Despite this being a five-year course, everyone does a research-based BMedSci (Hons) degree in year 3. The exam results of the first two years contribute 50% of the final degree mark. Students who leave the course after this have the benefit of a degree qualification, which they would not necessarily have at another medical school. This is a comfort, but not many students leave mid course. Many students use their projects to publish scientific papers or present them at conferences. These projects often involve hard work but provide excellent analytical and self-directed learning skills for clinicals.

Special study modules and electives

The eight-week elective is at the end of all clinical attachments and final exams in year 5. Most people choose a mixture of work and play; a short report is expected from everyone. Earlier in year 5 there are two five-week long SSMs. The choices are good and Nottingham currently offers 30 SSM places throughout Europe.

Facilities

Library   The medical library is on the ground floor of the medical school; it is large and the staff are friendly. It is well stocked with core texts and journals, but can become busy around exam times. It opens until 11.15 pm weekdays, and during the day at weekends for most of the year.

Computers   IT facilities are good, with over 200 terminals in the medical school. There is unlimited and free access to email, the internet, teaching CD ROMs and computer-assisted learning packages for teaching and revision. The recently redesigned Networked Learning Environment allows internet access to lecture handouts, slides, and learning aids from outside the medical school. The main computer room is open 24 hours a day. Facilities at outlying hospitals are improving.

Clinical skills   This is a series of newly built rooms dedicated to teaching clinical skills such as examining patients. The laboratory is staffed and resources have rapidly grown to an excellent level. It is used on a casual basis and has many self-teaching aids – suturing practice kits, models of eyes, ears, arms (for blood pressure), videos, etc.

Welfare

Student support

As a whole the university has a friendly and open feel. Student welfare is taken very seriously. In the medical school every student is allocated a tutor who can address academic or personal problems. The students organise a mentoring system in which first-years are allocated individual second-year "parents". Whether or not you meet regularly with your "parent" depends on how well you get on; however, a high rate of adoption and incest leaves most people happy! The university and Students' Union have welfare, legal, financial, and counselling services, along with an active Niteline (night-time counselling service) run by students.

Accommodation

Almost all first-years are housed in good-quality university accommodation; these are mostly catered halls, though some students opt for self-catering flats. There are 12 medium-sized halls on the main campus, each with its own bar. A further three large halls are found on the newly built Jubilee campus, about 15 minutes' walk from the main campus or QMC. In subsequent years you can apply to stay in halls, though most students move into private rented houses: 80% choose to live in Lenton, which is a relatively safe student area 20 minutes' walk from the campus and town. House-hunting begins very early after Christmas; most students organise it themselves without university vetting. The Union organises house-hunting for first-years wanting to live out before their first term.

Placements

The teaching hospitals are all located within one rush-hour drive of Nottingham. The amount of hands-on experience, group sizes, and facilities tend to improve as the distance from the QMC increases. The smaller hospitals are generally friendlier, although more work is sometimes expected. Accommodation is provided free of charge in Mansfield.

Clinical visits in years 1 and 2 often require some travelling, but transport or suggested routes are provided. Clinical attachments are mostly in Nottingham at the QMC and Nottingham City Hospital (five miles), or a short distance away in Derby (15 miles) and Mansfield (20 miles). Students usually share car lifts and there are few problems with transport.

Sports and social

City life

The city centre is attractive, compact, and has good shopping facilities. Nottingham is renowned for its inexpensive and diverse bars, clubs, pubs, and restaurants. The theatres are good, but there are few live music venues. The city centre is within walking distance of most off-campus accommodation, and a 10-minute bus ride (£1) from campus. Because of its central location travel to most other cities is quick and easy. The Peak District and surrounding countryside provide a welcome escape where students can risk life and limb far away from biochemistry revision.

Uni life

Student life is rich and varied, and there is plenty of time to enjoy it while doing a medical degree. The student medical society (MedSoc) provides a good range of social events, balls, and guest lectures. There are hundreds of university clubs and societies facilitating much interaction within the student body, notably CockSoc (cocktails, not male chickens or anything else!). Nottingham has one of the largest student rags in the country, called 'Karni'. This raises about £230 000 for charity from activities in the first term. On-campus entertainment revolves around hall life, and includes bars and themed parties. In later years the pub and club scenes of Lenton and the city dominate. MedSoc organises many cocktail parties, guest lectures and other social events.

The main distinguishing feature of Nottingham medics' social life is the extent to which medical students are mixed with the whole university population. After the first year many medics live with their non-medic friends from halls. Lenton, the main student area, is well equipped with cheapish pubs, launderettes, late-opening shops, take-aways, video rental shops, and buses. Although the campus accommodation is excellent, the university could take more responsibility for off-campus housing.

Sports life

Nottingham has good-quality, accessible sporting facilities. Medics' teams play against the hall teams; they are particularly strong in hockey, rugby, tennis, and football. Most sports and standards of ability are represented somewhere in the university. The clubs provide a focus for excellent social lives.

Great things about Nottingham

- You get a bonus degree (BMedSci) without having to do an extra year; this is very useful later in your career.
- Good social life for students, with variety, value, and accessibility along with many active and friendly student societies.
- Beautiful campus, with good community spirit and healthy interhall rivalry.
- Integration of medics with non-medics in halls broadens social circles and reduces the cliqueyness that medics are sometimes accused of!
- After the first year all your hall friends remain within walking distance by moving to the student area (Lenton).

Bad things about Nottingham

- Because of the poor Union bar and lack of a campus venue for top bands there is little to attract medics back to campus after their first year.
- It is felt that the university attracts students of a similar background, leading to a lack of diversity within the student population.
- House-hunting begins too early (January) and can be stressful.
- Experiences of the third-year Honours project are very variable in terms of workload, expectations, and assessment.
- The preclinical course is too lecture based.

Additional application information

Average A-level requirements	• AAB, including chemistry and biology. GCSE grade A in chemistry, biology, and physics, and grade B in English and maths. Six grade As required in total
Average Scottish Higher requirements	• AB in chemistry and biology at CSYS/Advanced Higher level, plus 2 grade Bs in Highers
Make-up of interview panel	• Two assessors (GPs, clinicians, academics)
Months in which interviews are held	• November–March
Proportion of overseas students	• 10%
Proportion of mature students	• 10%
Faculty's view of students taking a gap year	• Encouraged as long as experience is constructive
Proportion of students taking intercalated degrees	• All students do a BMedSci degree without doing an extra year
Possibility of direct entrance to clinical phase	• No
Fees for graduates	• £1100
Fees for overseas students	• £9660 pa (years 1+2) and £17 730 (years 3–5)
Assistance for elective funding	• Several grants available
Assistance for travel to attachments	• None from university
Access and hardship funds	• Yes
Weekly rent	• Halls £40 (self-catering) £95 (fully catered) Private £45–£50
Pint of lager	• Union bar £1.40 City centre pub £2.20
Cinema	• £3–£5
Nightclub	• Free–£4 Mon–Fri, though posh clubs charge more at the weekend

Further information

Admissions Officer
Faculty Office
Queen's Medical Centre
University of Nottingham
Nottingham NG7 2RD
Tel: 0115 970 9379
Fax: 0115 970 9922
Email: medschool@nottingham.ac.uk
Web: http://www.nottingham.ac.uk

Oxford

Key facts	Undergraduate course	Graduate course
Course length	6 years	4 years
Total number of medical students	677	20
Applicants in 2002	788	150
Interviews given in 2002	93% (100% of clinical)	
Places available in 2002	150	20
Places available in 2003	150	30
Entrance requirements	AAA	
Mandatory subjects	Chemistry	Biomedical science Honours degree
Male:female ratio	45:55	
Premed course	No	
Fast-track course	No	Yes

Oxford is a unique place. If you would like to live in either modern accommodation or 15th century halls and meet students of all backgrounds; have the double benefits of a small college and a large university; with a traditional yet innovative medical course, then Oxford is for you!

As with most medical schools the course has undergone some recent changes and the size of the school is gradually being increased by 50%. The recent addition of an accelerated course for bioscience graduates is another innovation.

Some may criticise the lack of clinical involvement during the first three years of the six-year undergraduate course. However, the firm scientific basis of medicine is of vital importance and the acquisition of skills, such as the critical evaluation of papers and an understanding of research, is rightly given very high priority. Three years before significant patient contact may seem like a long time to some, but the knowledge and skills gained during the preclinical course will be of use for the rest of your career, and having an "extra" science degree is no bad thing when applying for medical jobs.

The course demands the very highest level of academic ability and commitment. However, your college tutor, who selects you in the first place, has a vested interest in your success and, in most cases, works very hard on your behalf – no-one is left to struggle. The short terms and long holidays also make the hard work survivable and enjoyable.

Education

Oxford Medical School was recently assessed by the QAA as a single six-year course, but for practical purposes there remains a clear-cut division between the preclinical and clinical courses in Oxford. At present, in the preclinical school the first five terms are spent studying the basic medical sciences (anatomy, biochemistry, physiology, pathology, and neuroscience), and the final four terms working for an Honours degree. (The timetable for the first two years is currently under review, but the subjects will remain the same.) Application to the clinical school is competitive, with about 55-65% of the Oxford preclinical students staying on. The rest go mainly to London or Cambridge, and there is an influx of students from elsewhere – mainly Cambridge – with additions from London and the Scottish medical schools.

The clinical course lasts three years and aims to deliver the best teaching of both scientific principles and clinical practice. It is in a particularly good position to do so, because of the combination of its small size and the very high quality of its academic and clinical staff. Year 4 consists of medicine, surgery, and an eight-week laboratory medicine course (pathology), together with a residential general practice attachment, ethics, and communication skills. Special study modules (SSMs) are an exciting and innovative addition to the fourth year. These can be taken in subjects such as philosophy, theology, chronic illness, and creativity, where students are free to explore their interests. The year begins with an improved five-week foundation course, a fortnight of which is dedicated to teaching from year 6 students. This allows a gentle transition from preclinical to clinical studies for the year 4 students while giving the final-years a chance to teach.

Year 5 contains all the specialist rotations: paediatrics, obstetrics and gynaecology, A&E, orthopaedics, general practice, neurology, ENT, ophthalmology, and psychiatry. Year 6 focuses again on medicine and surgery (five weeks each), with a 10-week elective period, 14 weeks of clinical special study modules, a six-week PRHO shadowing at a district general hospital (DGH), and several revision weeks. Throughout the clinical course there is a great deal of ward-based teaching, with both consultants and the more junior doctors (all of whom are keen to practise being teaching hospital consultants!). The modular form of the specialist rotations means that there is no easy fifth year, but the pressure at finals is much reduced. At present, as almost all the clinical students are in Oxford at any one time there is a strong sense of group identity and a very full social life.

Teaching

In the preclinical years the basic medical sciences are taught by lectures and practicals, supported by most colleges giving tutorials with two to three students, two to three times a week.

Assessment

Currently, the assessments are at the end of the first year and before Easter in the second year, and consist of essay papers, short notes, and problem-solving questions. The practicals are assessed continuously and practical books must be kept up to date.

Intercalated degrees

All students spend the last terms of the preclinical phase working for an Honours degree in physiology or psychology (unless they are already graduates). The degree course has a large amount of flexibility, and students are encouraged to follow courses that interest them.

Special study modules and electives

There is a 10-week elective in the sixth year and most go abroad. Some of the colleges can help financially. The 14 weeks of SSMs in the final year are more clinical in nature than the modules of the first clinical year. There are over 60 options, ranging from the traditional (e.g. cardiology, anaesthetics, general practice) to the innovative (creativity in healthcare, medical publishing, medical anthropology, or even a language), and can be either purely clinical, research, or a mixture of both. If the extensive list does not cover the one subject that you desperately want to study, you are free, with the medical school's permission, to arrange your own.

Facilities

Library   Oxford is very well catered for with respect to libraries. At preclinical level, the Radcliffe Science Library (RSL) and college libraries are the most useful and used. College facilities vary but are in general good to excellent. The RSL has an incredible number of books and journals, but rather limited opening hours out of term. The Cairns Library is located at the John Radcliffe Hospital, and is the library used during clinical years. It is very well stocked and open 24 hours a day, 365 days a year.

Computers   The computing facilities are very good in colleges, departments, libraries and, at clinical level, in Osler House and the Cairns Library, where a large number of computers are reserved exclusively for medical students. Computer-assisted learning is soon to be introduced, and all lecture notes and resources for courses such as the laboratory medicine course are available electronically.

Clinical skills   A laboratory currently exists and is used for medical and surgical skills teaching. From next year a new larger laboratory is due to be built and will be used to teach a more comprehensive list of skills required for use as a PRHO. An automated dummy (called Harvey!) has also recently been purchased for skills teaching.

Welfare

Student support

Oxford students are clever yet friendly and very social. There is a niche for everyone. The university tutoring system works well in the preclinical years because of the collegiate system. In clinical years, when links with the college are not as strong, the system does not work so well but is supplemented by good support, be it academic or pastoral, from the medical school. Colleges provide significant financial assistance, ranging from subsidised accommodation, meals and entertainment, to elective funding and hardship grants. Oxford University has welfare and counselling facilities, in addition to the provision by the medical school and colleges.

At preclinical and especially clinical levels medical students tend to know each other very well. Depending on your viewpoint, this can either be an advantage or a disadvantage, but most seem to enjoy the camaraderie and banter, whether in the bar or in the dissection room! One of the great things about Oxford is the collegiate system: this broadens your horizons and makes it very easy to make friends with non-medics. At the clinical level, Osler House Club (the Students' Union) provides a very relaxed way of meeting people and making friends.

Accommodation

Preclinical students will find their life completely integrated with that of students in other subjects and will live with them in college accommodation. Many of the college buildings are old and beautiful, but do bear in mind that sometimes the accommodation you will actually live in will either be 1950s or private lodgings. All the accommodation is of a reasonable to good or excellent standard, and fairly cheap.

Things are very different for clinical students, however. Very few live on college sites, as the majority of graduate accommodation is in nearby annexes. The exception is Green College, which was established for medical students and is still largely populated by them. Many prefer to live out during their clinical training, as it affords more independence than college can provide, and there is plenty of good-quality private accommodation in Oxford.

Placements

The early years are spent studying basic medical sciences in and around the centre of Oxford. This is amid the Oxford colleges, with their long traditions of study and learning. The clinical school is based at the John Radcliffe Hospital (JR), which is a large teaching hospital situated in Headington, two miles east of Oxford city centre and easily accessible by bus or bike. It is modern, large, and contains all of Oxford's acute medical and surgical services. The Churchill Hospital is increasingly becoming a specialist centre for certain services, such as transplants, oncology, and soon diabetes and endocrinology. The Radcliffe Infirmary contains services for neurology, ENT, ophthalmology, and plastic surgery. It is due to be closed down and relocated to the JR site within the next five years. The Nuffield Orthopaedic Hospital, the Warneford and Littlemore psychiatric hospitals are smaller centres used for specific modules of the course. All the hospitals are easily reached by bike, bus, or car (although parking is almost impossible!).

Although other hospitals in Banbury, Reading, Swindon, Northampton, and Bath are used, the majority of a student's time will still be spent in Oxford. Many find this very useful, as it allows them to be involved in university and college life, whether sports, drama, music, or other activities. There are, however, ample opportunities to travel (in addition to the elective) for those who want to: for example, several of the specialties (such as paediatrics, and deliveries in obstetrics) can be studied in other parts of the country or world.

Sports and social

City life

Oxford, the "city of dreaming spires", is a small city with easy access to the rest of the country, and London in particular (only 50 minutes by train and 90 minutes by coach). Many preclinical students survive the first three years without needing to travel more than five minutes on foot from the centre of the city, but at clinical school you are forced to move a little further afield. The town centre has the usual core of shops, and you will find it sufficient for most needs. Having said that, it doesn't compare to most "real" cities for variety. Culturally there is a lot going on, particularly if you like theatre and music. It has to be said that the club scene in Oxford is not very exciting and wouldn't suit the more dedicated punter, but you can get to and from London on buses leaving every 12–15 minutes, 24 hours a day.

Uni life

There are numerous university- and college-based clubs and societies dedicated to ensuring that students get the most they can out of their time in Oxford. At preclinical level these often form a prominent part of most people's social life, with the medical society (MedSoc) supplementing this. The societies range from the sublime to the ridiculous, and you will find that talents you never realised you had are catered for.

The clinical school social life tends to revolve around Osler House, a 1920s house in the grounds of the John Radcliffe run for and by clinical students. There is a bar, a television room, computing facilities, pool table, and a pleasant garden, with lunch served daily. The Osler Committee organises many events – social, sporting, and cultural. However, many clinical students also remain involved in other aspects of university life, be it at their college or elsewhere. The clinical school pantomime, *Tingewick*, deserves a special mention. This occurs every year and is a great chance for the students to get their own back at their consultants and anyone else who deserves parody.

Sports life

Oxford is famous for its rowing and rugby, but other sports are well represented too. In particular, the collegiate structure means that there are both facilities and opportunities for involvement in sport at any level of ability. All the colleges have sports pitches and boat houses, and many can provide squash and tennis courts as well. Intercollegiate competitions (Cuppers) form one focus for the competitive energy, and the very committed will find themselves competing at the highest levels – the Varsity competitions. Even if you lack speed, strength, skill, accuracy, or talent in general, you will still be able to find a team of your level and skill! In the collegiate events the clinical school is represented by the Osler–Green teams, who regularly manage to field competitive sides.

Good things about Oxford 👍

- The collegiate system – meeting students in a variety of subjects, which predisposes to broader interests and education.
- Tutorial system: having one to one or two to one tuition, with the academic support that this offers. Consequently, very few students fall behind in their work.
- The influx of up to 50 new students from other medical schools in the fourth year creates a fantastic opportunity to make new friends when you begin your clinical training.
- Excellent scientific and clinical teaching, together with a stimulating environment in a university with a first-class, worldwide reputation.
- Oxford is a beautiful city in which to work and, together with its traditions, this makes Oxford a unique and rare experience.

Bad things about Oxford 👎

- The public perception of Oxford is behind the times and relies too much on stereotypes. These are inaccurate and unhelpful – don't be discouraged from applying!
- Some students at Oxford are incredibly hard working, so the pressure can build up at times.
- The scientific nature of the course, particularly during the preclinical years, does not suit everyone.
- The nightlife in Oxford is limited, but London is nearby and easily reached.
- The PRHO matching scheme doesn't work well.

Additional application information

Average A-level requirements	• AAA, including chemistry
Average Scottish Higher requirements	• Five A grades and CSYS or A-level passes (including chemistry)
Make-up of interview panel	• Preclinical: one or two college Fellows (may be several interviews). Clinical: panel of four, including clinicians, preclinical teacher, and at least one woman
Months in which interviews are held	• Preclinical: December. Clinical: late Jan/early Feb
Proportion of overseas students	• 4% (preclinical) 7% (clinical)
Proportion of mature students	• 4–6%
Faculty's view of students taking a gap year	• Generally supportive if for good reasons, but consult individual college admission tutors
Proportion of students taking intercalated degrees	• 100% – the Honours degree is an integral part of the course
Possibility of direct entrance to clinical phase	• Yes (Honours graduates only) with preclinical qualifications undertaken in the UK
Fees for overseas students	• £9975 pa (preclinical) £18 285 pa (clinical) Non-EU students pay college fees of £1500–£3500
Assistance for elective funding	• Very helpful financially and otherwise. Colleges also have funds
Assistance for travel to attachments	• Yes
Access and hardship funds	• Available, especially if unforeseen circumstances cause hardship
Weekly rent	• Halls vary, but normally less than the private sector. Private £60
Pint of lager	• Union bar £1–£1.50 City centre pub £1.80–£2.50
Cinema	• £3.50–£4.50
Nightclub	• Free–£7

Further information

Oxford Colleges Admission Service
The University Offices
Wellington Square
Oxford OX1 2JD
Tel: 01865 270207
Fax: 01865 270208
Web: http://www.ox.ac.uk

Clinical Medical School Offices
John Radcliffe Hospital
Headington
Oxford OX3 9DU
Web: http://www.medicine.ox.ac.uk/medsch

Peninsula (Exeter and Plymouth)

Key facts	Peninsula
Course length	5 years
Total number of medical undergraduates	127 (proposed 800)
Applicants in 2002	First intake September 2003
Interviews given in 2002	
Places available in 2002	127
Places available in 2003	167
Entrance requirements	340 points from 3 A-levels
Mandatory subjects	1 science subject
Male:female ratio	–
Premed course	No
Fast-track course	No

As part of the expansion of medical school places in the UK the government has sanctioned the opening of several new schools. One of the new institutions is the product of collaboration between the Universities of Exeter and Plymouth, and is called the Peninsula Medical School. The following is a statement from the School.

The Peninsula Medical School – one of the first new medical schools in this country for nearly 30 years – opened its doors to students for the first time in October 2002. The school has been formed through a unique partnership between the Universities of Exeter and Plymouth and the NHS in Devon and Cornwall to offer the Bachelor of Medicine, Bachelor of Surgery (BmBs) degree programme.

As well as being new in the physical sense, Peninsula is also very new in its approach to medical training, as the school's Dean, Professor John Tooke, explains: *'This is a time of change in the National Health Service. There will be an increasing emphasis placed on health services within the community setting and less obvious divisions between primary and secondary care. The patient of the future will receive care from teams of healthcare professionals working together.'*

What is so special about our course is that, because it is new we are unhampered by any existing structures, we can design it around the latest health service plans to produce doctors equipped to rise to the challenges that lie ahead.

What this means is that tomorrow's doctors are likely to have a far wider understanding of all aspects of patient care. From week 1 of the BMBS course, students will spend time in the community developing their clinical skills – learning from GPs, nurses, and other healthcare professionals as they go about their daily working lives. This practical experience of working as part of a team is seen as crucially important in a modernised health service that aims to put the patient, rather than bureaucracy, at the heart of future strategic planning.

One hundred and twenty-seven students commenced their BMBS degree in October 2002. This figure rises to 167 in 2003, and by 2007 the school will be training approximately 800 new doctors. Interviews for the 2003 intake began in November 2002 and offers will be made to successful applicants in early 2003.

The Peninsula Medical School experience
- Learning opportunities are provided in a variety of healthcare environments in the south west, from general practice to specialist hospitals.
- The focus on clinical skills training means students will undertake practical clinical work from the first week of the course.
- Students will experience the best educational practices in a research-rich environment and will benefit from a problem-based learning approach, studying with leading medical educators.
- Clinical problems will be approached holistically to ensure students appreciate the personal and social dimensions, in addition to the biomedical basis and the importance of multiprofessional teamwork in the delivery of contemporary healthcare.

For more information about the Peninsula Medical School please ring 01752 764261 or visit the Web at: http://www.pms.ac.uk.

Additional application information

Average A-level requirements	• 340 points from 3 A-levels – 1 science and preferably 1 non-science related subject
Average Scottish Higher requirements	• 340 points from 5 Highers; AAAAB in both science and non-science subjects
Make-up of interview panel	• 3 panellists from healthcare professional and community backgrounds
Months in which interviews are held	• November/December
Proportion of overseas students	• First intake September 2003
Proportion of mature students	• First intake September 2003
Faculty's view of students taking a gap year	• Deferment is allowed provided it is stated on application. Usually deferment for one year only is permitted
Proportion of students taking intercalated degrees	• N/A
Possibility of direct entrance to clinical phase	• N/A

Further information

Email: medadmissions@pms.ac.uk
Web: http://www.pms.ac.uk, http://www.exeter.ac.uk, http://www.plymouth.ac.uk

Royal Free and University College London

Key facts	Royal Free
Course length	6 years
Total number of medical undergraduates	1840
Applicants in 2002	2300 +
Interviews given in 2002	c. 1100
Places available in 2002	330
Places available in 2003	330
Entrance requirements	ABB
Mandatory subjects	Chemistry plus biology at A or AS-level
Male:female ratio	45:55
Premed course	No
Fast-track course	No

One of the largest medical schools in the UK lies in an exciting, attractive and vibrant part of London. The Royal Free and University College London Medical School (RFUCMS) is the product of the recent merger of two world-class institutions: Royal Free Hospital School of Medicine (Hampstead) and University College London Medical School (Bloomsbury). Our parent schools have excellent reputations for teaching and research and include a number of world-famous institutions. These include the Institute of Child Health (Great Ormond Street), the Institute of Neurology (the National Hospital for Neurology and Neurosurgery), the Institute of Laryngology and Otology, and the Institute of Ophthalmology (Moorfields Eye Hospital). RFUCMS offers a modern course, taught by respected academics and clinicians, as well as some very friendly students.

Education

The new curriculum started in 2000. It is a six-year integrated systems-based course, including an intercalated BSc for non-graduates. Clinical experience starts from day 1, although the preclinical/clinical divide has not entirely been abandoned.

Teaching

The core curriculum is arranged into three distinct phases. Phase I consists of sequential systems-based learning modules which cover all basic medical subjects. Phase II (science and medical practice, years 3 and 4) consists of a series of sequential clinical attachments, reflecting and building on the systems-based modules of Phase I. In year 3 there are two half-days of formal teaching (including basic science) each week. In year 4 there are blocks of formal teaching (again including basic science) between clinical attachments. In Phase III (professional development, year 5) there are clinical attachments in general practice, accident and emergency and district general hospitals, as well as selective specialist clinical attachments and a period of elective study.

Running throughout these sequential modules for all five years of the course there are three vertical modules: mechanisms of drug action/use of medicines; society and the individual; and pathology. There is also a continuous strand of professional development from year 1 through to year 5.

Assessment

Assessment includes MCQs, OSCEs, and oral examinations. It is integrated with a considerable amount of formative assessment and a portfolio of coursework that must be completed to a satisfactory standard in order to permit entry to end-of-year summative assessments, which determine progression.

Intercalated degrees

All non-graduate students are expected to complete an intercalated BSc. Although the majority of students will intercalate between Phases I and II, some will choose to do so later in the medical degree programme, especially if they wish to pursue a BSc programme designed for students with greater clinical experience. The range of subjects to choose from is impressive and new intercalated BSc course units and degree programmes in 2002 were extended to include medical ethics and law, forensic archaeology, and space physiology and medicine. Information on the intercalated BSc is given to students in their second year.

Special study modules and electives

In addition to the core curriculum there are special study modules to permit the study of selected aspects in depth. These may be medical or non-medical and can include law, history of medicine, arts and modern languages. Four must be taken in Phase I, three in Phase II and two in Phase III. A period of elective study is taken in the final year and most students choose to spend this abroad. Limited funding is available.

Facilities

Library   There are large medical and clinical science libraries on the Gower Street campus, a well-stocked and spacious library on the Royal Free campus, and a new and well-stocked library on the Archway (Whittington Hospital) campus. In addition, the many postgraduate medical institutes associated with UCL have specialist libraries within easy walking distance of Gower Street. The British Museum is a stone's throw away from the Gower Street campus as is the Wellcome Institute, the Institute of Neurology, the School of Pharmacy and the London School of Hygiene and Tropical Medicine.

Computers   There are clusters of networked computers throughout all RUMS campus sites and in many halls of residence. When they are not booked for formal teaching, students have free access on a first-come first-served basis. Most networked computers are Windows PCs, although there are some Apple computers. All students have free internet and email access and free printing resources, as well as a wide variety of networked software. IT skills are assessed at the beginning of the course, and there is a scheme for peer tutoring.

Clinical skills   There are clinical skills laboratories on all three "home" campuses, and in addition to timetabled sessions, students may arrange access at other times. They are all well liked by students, allowing such diverse activities as suturing sponges, cannulating plastic arms and catheterising plastic penises.

Welfare

Student support

In Phase I all students are assigned a personal tutor/academic adviser, normally a basic scientist who oversees their personal and academic development and provides pastoral care. In Phases II and III students are assigned personal tutors who are clinically qualified. In addition, the faculty tutorial team provide regular "walk-in surgeries", and most academic staff in UCL have an open-door policy or clearly advertised hours when they are available to students. UCL has a wide range of welfare, support and counselling services available for students.

Student feedback on course quality and teaching is actively sought through questionnaires, faculty education committees and staff–student consultative committees. Courses will be changed in the light of (valid) student comments. Organisation is generally very good, with comprehensive lecture notes being provided by lecturers. Lectures and formal tutorials still form an important part of the new course.

Accommodation

Practically all first-year students stay in UCL or University of London halls. Halls are generally acceptable, and a second year in halls is normally available during the BSc or final year. The accommodation office at Senate House offers help and legal advice to London students. To find better-value accommodation, many students choose to travel into central London from places like Finsbury Park and Camden.

Placements

The Royal Free and University College medical schools are on three main campuses. The Gower Street campus in Bloomsbury incorporates the faculties of life sciences and clinical sciences and has among its clinical facilities University College Hospital and the Middlesex Hospital. Most teaching in Phase I is based on the main Bloomsbury campus of UCL. The Wolfson Institute for Biomedical Research is a major development that was opened by the Princess Royal in April 2000 and the building houses new teaching facilities for medical students.

The campus in Hampstead is part of the Royal Free Hospital and a wide range of academic departments (including the Centre for Health Informatics and Multiprofessional Education) are based there. The Archway campus in Highgate is the site of the Department of Primary Care and Population Science. There is a further campus at the Whittington Hospital. Clinical teaching also takes place in many associated university district hospitals and in a range of general practice and community settings.

Most clinical teaching placements outside the university are at UCL/Middlesex, Royal Free and Whittington Hospitals, all of which are in central London. District general hospital attachments are normally in outer London (Barnet, Northwick Park, Stanmore, North Middlesex), or further afield (for example Stoke-on-Trent, Truro, King's Lynn and Northampton). A new skyscraping UCH is due to open around 2005 to replace the current UCH and Middlesex Hospitals.

Sports and social

City life

UCL's central London location places students very close to some of the finest theatres, concert halls and museums in the world. The Royal Free campus has both the cosmopolitan atmosphere of Hampstead and the green scenery of Hampstead Heath. In nearby Camden there are opportunities to see live music and visit Camden Lock market. The famous areas of Soho and Covent Garden are only a short walk away from the Gower Street campus.

Uni life

Students of the medical school are, like all UCL students, members of University College London Union, and they enjoy all the facilities and services that the Union provides. Medical students form a very large group within the total student population, and their special needs are provided for by medical student Union Officers on all three sites. As a community we call ourselves 'RUMS' (Royal Free and University College Medical Students).

The family-like community of medical students here is encouraged from day 1, when freshers are given a second-year "parent" to guide them through the first months of medical student life. Throughout the year the RUMS officers organise various events, including balls, theme nights and shows, beginning with the 14-day extravaganza of RUMS freshers' fortnight. As well as organising a Rag week and running more than 30 clubs and societies, the RUMS officers also represent medical students to the school on educational and welfare-related issues.

Medical students have their own bar/clubhouse in Huntley Street on the Gower Street campus, as well as social and Union facilities at the Royal Free campus. In addition, there is the main UCL Union, with centres on the Gower Street campus and in the Windeyer Building (part of the Middlesex Hospital site, a few minutes' walk from Gower Street). The excellent University of London Union (ULU) is directly adjacent to the Gower Street campus. This means there is an unparalleled variety of sports and social facilities available, with opportunities to meet students from other disciplines.

Your motto will become "work hard, play hard" and there is something for every RFUCMS student to enjoy: we have our own medic societies as well as the hundreds of Union societies to choose from. We also have our traditional medics' "comedy" revue company, which puts on an annual Christmas show for the benefit of the Middlesex Hospital, not to mention our legendary balls, together with the official Union entertainment. All dramatic, musical and operatic performances are shown in the college's own renowned West End venue on campus, the UCL Bloomsbury.

One of the most anticipated events is rag week, which is an orgy of money collecting for charity. You'll get up at 5 am to shake a tin at a tube station and go to bed at 3 am having exhausted yourself at a party or pub crawl. These weeks are a massive event in the social calendar that we all look forward to. The societies organise social events ranging from "civilised" dinners to rather less civilised initiations, and put on plays and musical shows alongside gigs and choral performances. Don't forget that at RUMS you are not confined to socialising within the medical school – you also have the varied clubs and societies of UCL to explore. RUMS really do get twice the fun of your average student!

Sports life

You can play for RUMS in most sports, but you are also entitled to play for the UCL Union and UL teams if you wish. They all compete in both national and local competitions in most sports. RUMS teams play at two sports grounds: one is in Enfield and the other is in Shenley, Hertfordshire. The latter is a 60-acre site catering for most sports and is the home ground of the UCL Union teams. The Enfield sports ground has been used for the summer ball in recent years, in addition to hosting the majority of the RUMS fixtures, and is widely regarded as our home ground. We have a very strong tradition of water-based sports. We row from the University boat house in Chiswick. One highlight of the sporting year is the United Hospital Bumps for eights on the Thames. The swimming pool in the basement of John Astor House is available to medical students, as are the weights room, gym, squash courts and billiards rooms. Somers Town Sports Centre is a new and important venue for UCL sports which is situated near the Bloomsbury campus. It offers excellent facilities for a number of the RUMS teams, including the basketball, netball, hockey and football clubs. The Union also provides an impressive gym complex, the Bloomsbury Fitness Centre. Finally, UCL students have full access to ULU facilities and societies and there is a large swimming pool, jacuzzi and sauna in the nearby Malet Street buildings. Of special interest are the various United Hospital sports clubs in which all members of our students' society are encouraged to participate.

Great things about RFUCMS

- One of the top-ranking universities in the UK for research in basic medical sciences and clinical medicine, with a school truly integrated into the multi-faculty institution of UCL with all the associated benefits in terms of sporting, cultural and social facilities.
- UCL's central London location places RFUCMS students very close to some of the finest theatres, concert halls and museums in the world. The Royal Free campus has both the cosmopolitan atmosphere of Hampstead and the green scenery of Hampstead Heath.
- Plenty of opportunity to mix socially and academically with non-medics at a multi-faculty university with many BSc opportunities.
- A major centre of biomedical research, with opportunities to work alongside world leaders in research at a school renowned for its teaching system, with plenty of small-group tutorials, a superbly equipped dissection suite and new teaching and learning facilities.
- RFUCMS medics are members of their own Union, the UCL Union and the University of London Union, so there is no shortage of student activity even though the opportunities of central London are on your doorstep.

Bad things about RFUCMS

- Central London can be a little daunting at first if you're not used to living in a big city; and crossing Euston Road every day can't be good for your health with its combination of pollution and dangerous drivers!
- The need to travel around London to get to different campuses: Gower Street (UCH), Archway (Whittington) and Hampstead (Royal Free), and the fact that you probably won't be able to avoid a 20-minute tube journey into college after you leave halls, unless you're lucky or rich!
- Living in London is only as expensive as you make it, but the rent is ridiculous. Expect to pay £100 a week.
- In a class of 330 it can be easy to be isolated and not meet all of your fellow students, especially in the early years. And as UCL is a 16 000-strong college you can feel like a very small fish in a very large pond when you first arrive.
- The visible signs of poverty, such as the homeless on the streets, can be depressing.
- Tough retake policy; for example in year 1 students must pass a further three papers with an overall pass of 50%, rather than resitting the one paper as with many other medical schools.

Average A-level requirements	• ABB, must include chemistry + pass in additional A or AS-level. Biology required to A or AS-level
Average Scottish Higher requirements	• Please check with the school
Make-up of interview panel	• Three (2–3 staff and/or one other – GP, medical student, head teacher)
Months in which interviews are held	• November–March
Proportion of overseas students	• 7%
Proportion of mature students	• 12%
Faculty's view of students taking a gap year	• Very positive, encouraged
Proportion of students taking intercalated degrees	• Compulsory (graduates exempted)
Possibility of direct entrance to clinical phase	• Oxbridge only
Tuition fees per year	• £1100
Fees for self-funding students	• n/a
Fees for graduates	• n/a
Fees for overseas students	• £13 495 preclinical £20 450 clinical
Assistance for elective funding	• Advice on funds available from registry
Assistance for travel to attachments	• Yes, for travel outside zone 2
Access and hardship funds	• Yes, some available
Weekly rent	• Halls £48–£120 Private £80+
Pint of lager	• Union bar £1.40 City centre pub £2.20
Cinema	• £3.50–£10
Nightclub	• Free–£20

Further information

Dr B Cross
Faculty Tutor
Faculty of Life Sciences
UCL
London WC1E 6BT
Tel: 020 7679 5467/5493
Email: medicaladmissions@ucl.ac.uk
Web: http://www.ucl.ac.uk/medical school

Students' Union: Medical Students' and Sites' Officer
25 Gordon Street
London WC1H 0AY
Tel: 020 7679 7949
Email: mss.officer@ucl.ac.uk
Web: http://www.uclu.org.uk

St Andrew's

Key facts	St Andrew's
Course length	3 years (preclinical only)
Total number of medical undergraduates	320
Applicants in 2002	492
Interviews given in 2002	Graduates, mature and access applicants normally interviewed, along with 10% of borderline applicants
Places available in 2002	112
Places available in 2003	112
Entrance requirements	ABB
Mandatory subjects	Chemistry
Male:female ratio	49:51
Premed course	No
Fast-track course	No

Established in the 15th century, St Andrew's is the oldest university in Scotland. It is set in a small picturesque town on the east coast of Fife. The course lasts for three years, during which the importance of the traditional preclinical subjects is emphasised. After this the vast majority of students head south for Manchester, where they complete their clinical studies (a further three years). The uniqueness of such a course provides a great opportunity for students to experience studying both in an ancient university town and in a big vibrant city. The faculty is small and students socialise with medics and non-medics alike.

Education

St Andrew's is the oldest university in Scotland, which explains the traditions and customs that surround being a student here. The course is quite traditional, being departmentalised rather than integrated, but it is frequently reviewed and improved to suit the needs of a modern doctor in training. The first two years are spent learning anatomy, physiology, cellular and molecular medicine, and behavioural sciences. A first-aid course is also completed in the first year. Second-year students also choose an SSM in the second semester, which is usually in the form of a project, as well as completing a course called Assessing Medical Evidence, covering skills in numeracy, critical thinking, experimental design, and evidence-based medicine. The third year is spent studying microbiology, pharmacology, pathology, public health, applied medical science, and behavioural sciences.

Students graduate in medical sciences, and then progress to a clinical school for a further three years before graduating as a doctor. There is a guaranteed place at Manchester and the vast majority go there, but students are at liberty to apply to another school for their clinical studies. The course still has a very traditional preclinical feel. There is little patient contact, although clinical relevance is always emphasised. The small class size for tutorials and dissection gives a great opportunity to develop good relationships between students and with staff. Some aspects of the course mimic the problem-based learning approach in operation at Manchester, and integration between the two schools has improved greatly over the last few years. One of the benefits of the course structure at St Andrew's is that students leave here with a degree whether or not they continue medical studies.

Teaching

Teaching is by lectures, tutorials, and practicals, with some tutorials using computer-based teaching. Anatomy is taught using cadavers, which the students dissect.

Assessment

Exams are varied and often include a mixture of MCQs, short-answer questions, essays, case studies, and vivas.

Intercalated degrees

An intercalated year is possible at the end of the third year for those who wish to convert their BSc into an Honours degree. Approximately 20% stay on for this additional year, including most of those who wish to apply to medical schools other than Manchester for their clinical studies.

Special study modules and electives

The electives are taken at the clinical school you attend. A special study module takes place in the second year. Opportunities for studying modules in subjects such as philosophy, ethics, pastoral care, and counselling exist, as well as more scientific areas such as histology.

Facilities

Library Opening hours are: Monday to Thursday 9 am–10 pm, Friday to Saturday 9 am–6 pm, and Sunday 1 pm–7 pm. A reasonable range of books is available, but many students buy the core texts because of the restricted availability of some titles.

Computers There are several computer rooms available and halls of residence have computer facilities. The university runs a 24-hour service in computer laboratories scattered around town.

Clinical skills Access to the laboratory is good and the staff are helpful.

Welfare

Student support

This is an area of major strength at St Andrew's. In such a small town the medics are well integrated into the university, and you will have the chance to get to know everyone at the school and make friends outside the faculty. The Dean and faculty are good and very supportive, and tend to get to know everyone by name quite quickly. The Students' Union provides welfare and counselling services, including a "Nightline" service for stressed students. The locals tend to be student friendly, if only because the university is the biggest local employer and we almost outnumber the locals. However, when the revelry surrounding some of the ancient traditions still upheld by the university gets a bit over the top, town and gown relations can become a little strained.

Accommodation

All students can spend their first year in university accommodation (halls and flats), and there are often rooms available for further years. Rooms are often shared and the standard of flats is generally good. Some halls are better than others, but none are bad. Other privately owned accommodation is available, over which the university has no control, and rents average £55–80 a week. Parking is difficult if you want to live in the town centre. There is a housing office at the university, which can help you find places.

Placements

The medical school consists mainly of the Bute Medical Building, referred to by students as "The Bute". Some other buildings in St Andrew's may be used, but they are all within walking distance of each other. St Andrew's is very small for a university town, so there is no problem getting around.

Students are attached to a local GP clinic in the second year for only a day, and there are also two hospital visits as part of the course in the third year. As part of the behavioural sciences course students are attached, in pairs, to a local family, whom they interview throughout the three years. Patient contact in St Andrew's is virtually non-existent: it is a true preclinical course.

For clinical placements, see the Manchester chapter.

Sports and social

City life

St Andrew's is a beautiful coastal town with a population of less than 20 000, and is famed for its golf. Being the oldest of Scotland's four ancient universities, it has more than its share of traditions and some of the oldest student societies. The students all live very near the centre of town, so it is never far to walk to meet a friend. There is a very good atmosphere among the students, with plenty of chances to mix with medics and non-medics, and enough things going on in the town, at the Union and with the societies to keep you as busy as you want to be. Tourists and golf followers can make the town bustle a bit too much at times, but you can go celebrity spotting with some success.

The town has easily enough pubs, restaurants, and cafes to keep most people happy, but ravers and shopaholics will have to travel to Edinburgh or Dundee for some real action. Outdoor types have easy access to the Grampian Mountains, and the nearby sea and beaches can be good fun. There is no railway station at St Andrew's, the nearest being Leuchars, which has regular bus services, or taxis which are about £8.

Uni life

The Union is good – especially for freshers getting to know the place – and alcohol is reasonably cheap, but the club scene is lacking, with very few bands or comedians. There are buses weekly to nightclubs in Dundee, 30 minutes away, which offer clubbers the chance to visit some of the busiest clubs in Scotland. The price for these buses is £5, which includes entrance to the club and a bus back to St Andrew's. MedSoc (called "The Bute") has good socials, including a famed ball as well as a raucous revue. There are lots of different types of societies, from the very sensible to the downright silly. Social life tends to focus around balls and events run by these societies. There is normally something each and every week.

Sports life

Most sports are supported, especially hockey and rugby, and there is a medics' competition every year called the "Hypertrophy". Medical school teams do not play every week, and keen players often get involved with their hall teams or the main university clubs. Interhall competitions are also popular. The facilities have been improved in recent years, such as the gym and athletics union. There is no university swimming pool. It is, of course, golf heaven, with the Royal and Ancient offering excellent deals for students. Membership is around £100 a year, which includes the Old Course.

Great things about St Andrew's

- We have a great new MedSoc website: http://www.butemedics.com.
- Small year group and good integration with non-medics.
- An excellent preclinical course.
- St Andrew's has a great pub and coffee-shop culture.
- Golf – dirt-cheap membership on the best courses in Scotland.

Bad things about St Andrew's

- Limited patient contact and low clinical content to course work.
- No nightclubs, if you discount the Union.

- Not many shops – you will probably shop in your home town or travel to Dundee.
- It can get a bit cold at times.
- Relatively small student numbers can make it difficult to "get away from it all".

Additional application information

Average A-level requirements	• AAB at one sitting. Must include chemistry and one other science
Average Scottish Higher requirements	• AAABB, including chemistry and one other science
Make-up of interview panel	• Three to four staff, admissions tutor, clinicians and lecturers (including at least one representative of an ethnic minority and of both genders)
Months in which interviews are held	• December–March
Proportion of overseas students	• 8.5%
Proportion of mature students	• 10%
Faculty's view of students taking a gap year	• Time should be used constructively, although not necessarily with a medical emphasis
Proportion of students taking intercalated degrees	• 20%
Possibility of direct entrance to clinical phase	• No clinical school
Tuition fees per year	• £1100 (E, W and N1 students only)
Fees for graduates	• £2740
Fees for overseas students	• £12 300
Assistance for elective funding	• No elective during course at St Andrew's
Access and hardship funds	• Some support available (for example small interest-free loans)
Weekly rent	• Halls £40–£85 Private £55–£80
Pint of lager	• Union bar £1.50 City centre pub £2.20
Cinema	• £3.50
Nightclub	• Union nightclub (*Megabop*) £3

Further information

Admissions Office
79 North Street
St Andrew's
Fife KY15 9AJ
Tel: 01334 462150 (Schools Liaison Service); 01334 476161 (University admissions)
Fax: 01334 463395
Email: admissions@st-andrews.ac.uk
Web: http://www.st-andrews.ac.uk

St Bartholomew's and the Royal London

Key facts	St Bart's
Course length	5 years
Total number of medical undergraduates	1200
Applicants in 2002	c. 1900
Interviews given in 2002	892
Places available in 2002	254
Places available in 2003	Approx. 254
Entrance requirements	ABB
Mandatory subjects	Chemistry or biology
Male:female ratio	47:53
Premed course	No
Fast-track course	Yes from 2003

The medical school of St Bartholomew's and the Royal London is centred in London's East End, one of the capital city's most exciting areas. Home to a large number of ethnic groups, this area is a fascinating place to study medicine as a result of the varied needs of its communities.

St Bartholomew's is the oldest hospital in the world and is a centre of excellence for many specialist disciplines. The Royal London was the first medical school in England and will be the site of our new medical school building, which will be completed in 2004. Plans are also under way to build a 1000-bed student village at the Mile End campus.

The school strives to be progressive, and the 2003 intake will be the fifth year who will study the new 1999 curriculum, which has problem-based learning at its core and a greater emphasis on the integration of clinical and preclinical elements of medical training.

The combined school of St Bartholomew's and the Royal London is part of Queen Mary and Westfield College. We were the first school to complete the merger process, so most of the difficulties with this are now a thing of the past.

Education

A new curriculum started in 1999 and is centred on the technique of problem-based learning (PBL). This new approach involves a reduced number of lectures, and students are encouraged to find their own answers to clinical problems using textbooks, journals, and the internet. All students follow the same core course, and are then able to broaden their knowledge in areas of particular interest during special study modules (SSMs). The traditional preclinical/clinical divide is now less distinct, as the new course integrates basic medical, human, and clinical sciences from day 1 until graduation. Bart's and London students are placed with GPs and hospitals during the first two years.

Teaching

In the first two years of the course teaching is systems based, concentrating on "Systems in Health" for the first year and "Systems in Disease" for the second. There is a mixed approach, including lectures, PBL and workshop sessions, and all aspects of the body system, such as the cardiovascular system, are considered as an integrated whole. For the final three years teaching is hospital based, with a continued emphasis on self-directed learning. Courses in communication skills (using actors and videotaping) and ethics run throughout the five years. Dissection is no longer part of the core course, and anatomy is taught using computer-aided learning programs, anatomical models, and already dissected specimens. Those who wish to dissect may do this as an SSM. St Bartholomew's and the Royal London Hospitals are the home sites for clinical teaching.

Assessment

Summer exams are set for years 1–4 of the course, and with the new curriculum "big bang" final examinations are a thing of past. Assessment is continuous, with credit being given for performance in both tutorials and examinations. At the end of the fifth year students are assessed on their "competence to practise" as a PRHO and must pass an integrated paper and clinical exams.

Intercalated degrees

Both BSc and BMedSci courses are offered. Popular courses include neuroanatomy and medical science (BMedSci), but some students have studied anthropology, psychology, and even German, although this kind of choice is rare. Students can choose to stay at QMW or go to another college for this year. Fees are payable for the year, but some funding is available.

Special study modules and electives

There is a wide variety of SSMs available, including clinical, research, complementary medicine, and journalism. It is also possible for some students to spend three-month attachments at partner institutions in Europe. The elective lasts two to three months, starting after Christmas in the fifth year of the course. There are some existing arrangements with institutions in other countries, which can make for a more easily organised trip. Students can go almost anywhere as long as they can find themselves a supervisor.

Facilities

Library   There are three large libraries, one at each site. The two hospital libraries have wonderful architecture, history, and atmosphere. QMW is large and can occasionally be noisy during the daytime. Availability of books can be variable. Libraries are open 9 am–9 pm on weekdays, 9 am–4 pm on Saturdays. The QMW library is also open on Sundays. There are also two large pathology museums at the hospitals. Unfortunately, in light of the events at Alder Hey Hospital, access to these is now severely restricted.

Computers   The school is well equipped on all three sites. All computing facilities and functions are available and regularly updated. Computers are increasingly used for teaching and are available during library hours and from 10 am to 8 pm at weekends. The computer rooms at Bart's and QMW are open late. There are also computer facilities at South Woodford halls.

Clinical skills   The skills laboratory at Bart's is for use by both medical and nursing students. The clinical skills centre is available to everyone in the school. First-years learn clinical skills in an adapted ward at Mile End Hospital.

Welfare

Student support

On the first day of college, freshers are assigned a senior student to act as their "parent" and guide them through the first few weeks and beyond. "Parents" introduce their "children" to their friends, take them out to dinner, and offer advice on all issues, from simple things such as work to more complicated matters such as their love life. This makes for a lot of integration between students from different years. All students are allocated their own academic tutor; for personal and other problems they have use of a pastoral pool of sympathetic doctors and senior lecturers. The Medical and Dental Students' Association appoints a student as Welfare Officer, as does QMW College. Counselling is available within 24 hours at QMW College. Those with mental health problems can be seen in confidence by a consultant at another teaching hospital in a reciprocal arrangement with the school.

Accommodation

Students at Bart's and the London can spend two to three years of their studies in college accommodation. New first-year students choose whether they wish to live in Queen Mary College or University of London (intercollegiate) accommodation, and whether they wish to be catered for or to cook for themselves. Most first-years live in either Dawson Hall, which is an old Bart's residence, Floyer House at the Royal London, or South Woodford Hall. South Woodford is the cheapest and most social but is rather run down and a long way from Mile End. Dawson Hall is more modern, with very good facilities and in the centre of London. It allows students to self-cater, but is more expensive. Floyer House has recently been refurbished and is close to the Union. In central London, students from all colleges of the University of London live together in intercollegiate halls. These are also a 20-minute tube ride away from college. With all residences students should check whether or not rent is payable during holidays. The tube pass from South Woodford to Mile End costs approximately £45 per month with a student discount card.

Most senior students live in the East End in shared houses. Almost everyone lives within walking distance of the Royal London and QM sites. Property is slightly cheaper in east London than in other parts of the capital. The Griffin Community Trust provides cheap (approx. £50 per week), luxurious housing in a very special development incorporating housing for the elderly, a community centre, and flats for clinical students. Student residents spend an hour or two a week with their elderly neighbours and play bingo, watch videos, or just chat. Both students and elders say how much they gain from the experience.

Placements

The medicine course is based at three sites: Bart's, the London, and QMW, which are all within three miles of each other in the City and East End of London. They are easily accessible by tube, bicycle, and bus. The Medical Sciences department at QMW in Mile End is where the first two years are based. This site has good facilities, including the Students' Union shop, computer laboratories, and the ever popular 'E1' nightclub. The final three years are spent in hospital. Many of the district general hospitals used are in or close to the East End and accessible by bus or tube. Some are close enough to cycle to.

Students can expect to be sent to attachments outside the main teaching hospitals. Placements are in district general and other associated hospitals (accommodation is provided free). Destinations include Southend-on-Sea and the semi-military hospital at Frimley Park. GP attachments and SSMs can be arranged country-wide.

Sports and social 🏆

Uni life

The Medical and Dental Students' Association is thriving and provides social and sporting opportunities as well as welfare services for all. The two medical student bars at Bart's and the London hold regular discos and theme nights. Wednesdays (after sports matches) and Fridays are the big nights for going out. The summer ball at Bart's is popular, and there are smaller balls for freshers' week, rag week, and at Christmas.

Rag week is one of the prides of the college and students raked in over £150 000 last year from street collections, marathon running, bed-pushing, and a fashion show, ranking us as one of the most successful rags in the country. A large TV screen in the bar regularly shows the main sports events. Freshers' fortnight is equally popular, and a massive effort is made to welcome new students to the college.

There are over 30 clubs and societies run by the Association, which offer students the chance to develop new interests, meet people, play sport, and have a good time. Among the most active societies are: the Drama Society, which stages productions every term, including the infamous Christmas show, and goes to the Edinburgh Festival; the Asian Society; the Music Society, which includes the choir, orchestra, brass groups, and several bands. QMW has more clubs and societies if there are not enough at the medical school, or if you have a particular interest not catered for.

Student social life revolves around the Association/Union buildings at both Bart's and the London. The Medical Student President is head of the Medical and Dental Students' Association and takes a sabbatical year from his or her studies solely to represent and protect the interests of the medical and dental student community. The newly refurbished Association building at the London and the bar at Bart's are for use by medics, dentists, and their guests. In the London Association building there is a café-bar and bookshop. The official Association magazine, *M.A.D.*, comes out at least twice a term and reports on social, sporting, and other events. A large Students' Union is also available at QMW Mile End campus.

Sports life

The Association clubs cater for nearly all sporting interests and most welcome beginners. There is an off-site sports ground and swimming pools at both Bart's and the London Hospital. There are also gyms at Bart's, QMW College, and South Woodford Halls, and squash at Bart's and QMW, as well as tennis and badminton courts. Bart's and the London have an enthusiastic rowing club based on the River Lea. Hockey, water polo, women's football, and rugby have had good successes in recent years. The cricket club is legendary, with strong first and second teams which win titles most years.

Great things about Bart's and the London 👍

- A brand new course, innovative curriculum and teaching, as well as enthusiastic and approachable staff.
- All students and visitors agree that we are a very friendly community with a close-knit atmosphere. Students tend to have friends from all years, rather than just their own.

- Reasonable rents for shared houses, considering that we are in the centre of London, and everyone lives close to each other.
- There are good year-round events, and the Union bar opens with regular late licences.
- Diverse area, with a wide range of things to do and cultures to experience. The East End is very trendy, with new bars and restaurants opening all the time. The *Evening Standard* recently nominated Tower Hamlets as London's sexiest borough!

Bad things about Bart's and the London

- Local areas – we are surrounded by very deprived communities, and although this means good clinical experience and pathology subject matter, it can be a bit depressing and at times it is necessary to be wary, as students have been assaulted.
- Travelling – there is some travelling between sites required, and the rush hour lasts for hours.
- Little interaction with non-medical students, and some bad feeling between the medics and QMW students.
- London is such a massive place that it can take you some time to feel at ease with its vastness.
- Expense – living and studying in London is more expensive than elsewhere.

Additional application information	
Average A-level requirements	• Chemistry and biology at AS-level, plus another science at A-level
Average Scottish Higher requirements	• AAAAB with CSYS in either chemistry or biology at grade B
Make-up of interview panel	• Clinician, basic medical scientist, and clinical student
Months in which interviews are held	• November–March
Proportion of overseas students	• 13%
Proportion of mature students	• 21%
Faculty's view of students taking a gap year	• Very supportive if applicants have positive plans for the year
Proportion of students taking intercalated degrees	• 50%
Possibility of direct entrance to clinical phase	• Yes, for Oxbridge students
Fees for graduates	• £1100
Fees for overseas students	• £13 180 pa (preclinical) and £21 950 pa (clinical)
Assistance for elective funding	• Some
Assistance for travel to attachments	• No
Access and hardship funds	• College administers access-type funds
Weekly rent	• Halls £65–£100 Private £60+ (average £80)
Pint of lager	• Union bar £1.70 City centre pub £1.80–£2.50
Cinema	• £3.80
Nightclub	• £4

St Bartholomew's and the Royal London

Further information

Admissions Office
Queen Mary and Westfield College
Turner Street
London E1 2AD
Tel: 020 7377 7611
Fax: 020 7377 7612
Email: medicaladmissions@qmul.ac.uk
Web: http://www.smd.qmul.ac.uk

Open days: July

St George's

Key facts	Undergraduate course	Graduate entry
Course length	5 years	4 years
Total number of medical students	1005	140
Applicants in 2002	1551	830
Interviews given in 2002	4.7%	5.5%
Places available in 2002	190	70
Places available in 2003	190	70
Entrance requirements	ABB + B at AS-level	Degree + GAMSAT exam
Mandatory subjects	Chemistry and biology	Degree (any subject)
Male:female ratio	52:48	
Premed course	No	No
Fast-track course	No	Yes

St George's Hospital Medical School (SGHMS) is located in the heart of Tooting, in south London, five minutes' walk from Tooting Broadway Underground station. It is a very welcoming school, with plenty of atmosphere and a wide variety of clinical experience available. St George's Hospital itself is one of the largest teaching hospitals in Europe, situated in a heavily populated part of London with pressing health needs. It offers two medical degree programmes: an established five-year course and a very new graduate-only accelerated four-year course. As well as medics, there are nursing, midwifery, physiotherapy, radiography, and biomedical science students at St George's, all of whom mix well with staff to create a strong feeling of community within the hospital. It is this, in particular, that makes SGHMS a great place to study. Most will thoroughly enjoy the atmosphere, but at the very least all will appreciate it.

Education

The course lasts five years, with clinical experience starting with visits to GP surgeries in the first year. Since 1996 all new medical students have undertaken the new special study modules (SSMs) at St George's. The aim of the SSM programme is to allow students to study, in depth, areas of particular interest to them.

Teaching

The first year begins with the common foundation module, in which much of the teaching is shared by all the first-year healthcare courses (nurses, physios, radiographers, biomeds, etc.) for the first term. The rest of the medics' teaching is then divided into two core cycles: 1 and 2. In core cycle 1 (years 1 and 2) students study systems modules integrated with some clinical experience and undertake two SSMs. In core cycle 2 (years 3–5) students get general clinical experience in hospitals, GP surgeries, etc., along with some specialty clinical teaching and two more SSMs.

Assessment

Exams take place every term through years 1–4 and all contribute to the final MBBS qualification. The fifth year is exam free apart from finals in June! Assessment takes the form of written exams: MCQs (negatively marked), short-answer questions and the odd essay, and synoptic assessments and practical exams: OSCEs (clinical examinations) and OSPEs 'spotters' (e.g. anatomy).

Intercalated degrees

An intercalated BSc can be taken after the second, third, or fourth year. The later the degree is taken the more clinical in nature it can be. Study can be at St George's Hospital or other London colleges/medical schools (or further afield if you so desire), with a wide range of courses available – choices are not restricted to medical or science subjects.

Special study modules and electives

Students have to take four SSMs in total, but do not despair because there is the opportunity to take some of them abroad! The elective is in the fifth year and can also be taken overseas. It lasts for two months and help with funding is sometimes available.

Facilities

Library Library facilities are extensive, with about 40 000 books, 800 journals on current subscription, and a total of 77 000 journals available. Other facilities include interlibrary loans, photocopying, a large history and archive collection, and an audiovisual room with a large variety of video material.

Computers   There is an excellent range of computing facilities available, with networked database, CD-ROM, and interactive media. The library has a Unicorn catalogue for public access, over 100 workstations for network access, Word for Windows, and Excel; scanning facilities are also available. There is also a large 24-hour access computer room in the medical school (Windows and multimedia) with about 30 terminals. A computer room with eight computer stations is at the halls of residence.

Clinical skills   These facilities have been hugely improved in recent years, with an incredible range of realistic models for students to practise on before being faced with real patients. The rooms housing these gadgets are open 9 am–5 pm Monday to Friday, so students can walk in any time they have a free moment. In addition, the clinical skills facilitator is usually on hand to offer guidance on technique.

Welfare

Student support

Students at St George's tend to be very friendly and easy-going by nature. There is a strong school spirit and students are very supportive of each other. All freshers are assigned a "mother" or "father" student to look after them in their first year. There is normally no problem in borrowing lecture notes and getting useful advice. The school has counselling services locally, and students can use ULU (University of London Union) facilities.

Accommodation

In their first year students can live in hall, which, at only 15 minutes' walking distance from the school and costing only £57.50 per week, is possibly one of the best deals in London! There is a downside in that rooms are a bit on the small side, and baths, toilets, and kitchen facilities may have to be shared between six and eight people. 2003 will also see the construction of a new set of student accommodation, which will be bigger and better equipped. Tooting itself is filled with eager landlords waiting to accommodate local medical students, and rents in the area are more favourable than in many other parts of London.

Placements

The medical school is part of the main teaching hospital but occupies its own distinct area. There are six floors containing the library, computer rooms, teaching theatres, clinical laboratories, offices, and student area. The main hospital, including shop, canteen, and small bank branch (NatWest), is easily accessed from the medical school. On the second floor is the School Club (equivalent of a Students' Union). This comprises a bar, student offices, a coffee shop, school bookshop, games room, music room, and snooker room. Many students and staff go there to relax for lunch and coffee breaks, and many of the extracurricular activities are held there. There is also a student shop downstairs.

From the third year, students are placed at a variety of different other hospitals for specialty training. Much of the training (about three-quarters) will take place at St George's. There is usually a choice of where you go, travel expenses are reimbursed, and accommodation is free. Travel to hospitals other than St George's does not usually take more than half an hour to an hour by public transport. The distance to attachments increases in the final year, as you reach the end of your training. Most of the attachments are at least an hour or so by public transport, with the furthest being Darlington in the north of the country. Luckily, though, you are able to choose where you do these attachments, so you don't get stuck somewhere you don't want to be.

Sports and social

Uni life

St George's bar is one of the biggest and cheapest in the country, and is the scene of many a great night for many medical students. Discos and club nights are on alternate Friday nights, comedy nights and bands are well attended, and much fun is had by all. There is a wide-screen TV with satellite, films, and the main football and international rugby matches, etc. are regularly screened. There is a colossal range of societies and clubs to join, from all the conventional sporting ones like rugby and cricket to a parachuting club and a hill-walking society. There are various religious societies, the orchestra and musical societies, also a debating society – the list is endless. The School Club is very supportive of new clubs.

First and foremost, St George's is now the only free-standing medical school in the UK. The only other students around the place are in the caring professions or professions allied to medicine. There is a great feeling of camaraderie in the college: you will get to know most people in your year and many others. There is much mixing between year groups and with students of the other disciplines. This is partly because there are so many social events organised by the Students' Union. The medical school itself encourages students and staff to take as positive an attitude to their extracurricular interests as it does to studying.

Sports life

For the major outdoor sports St George's uses its own sports ground at Cobham, which is in Surrey. The rowing teams use the Boat House at Chiswick, where many other London colleges row. At the hospital itself is the Rob Lowe Sports Centre, which has six squash courts and two general fitness rooms with exercise bikes, treadmills, rowing machines, and step machines. There is also a weights room and a large sports hall for team sports, such as five-a-side football, and basketball. There are regular circuit training and aerobic lessons.

Great things about St George's

- Its small, close-knit community, with the best bunch of easy-going, fun-loving guys and girls you'll ever meet.
- The bar – now newly refurbished and the "best thing since sliced bread", according to the first-years. Definitely the heart and soul of the med school, and with ridiculously cheap beer to boot!

- Location, location, location! The med school is actually INSIDE one of the biggest teaching hospitals in Europe, giving easy access to loads of weird and wonderful pathologies, and making St George's one of the most renowned clinical teaching hospitals in the country. In some cases, if you do have to travel to a peripheral site expenses are reimbursed and accommodation provided.
- Really friendly staff and tutors ready to help you along your way, and if you do get stuck it is normally quite easy to find someone to help you out, be it academic or exam problems, clinical skills or personal stuff.
- Freshers' fortnight – yes, that's right, St George's offers two weeks of continuous freshers' events, from the principal's boat party to a three-legged pub crawl, to numerous random fancy dress discos and the Wimbledon pram race.

Bad things about St George's

- Although you are at a London medical school, St George's cannot pretend it is in central London. Tooting to Leicester Square is about 25 minutes on the tube and 30 minutes on the night bus.
- Lack of students studying anything apart from health sciences can limit the conversation a bit, to say the least!
- Parking at or near the hospital can be difficult and expensive.
- St George's does not have the capacity to offer an intercalated BSc to all its students, although most of those who do want to pursue this course of study usually manage it.
- The canteen can be overpriced and undercooked. There are plenty of cheap fried chicken, Indian and Chinese places to eat in Tooting, but there is a distinct absence of anything remotely healthy. However, with the newly built school shop, the variety on offer has been hugely increased in the last year.

Additional application information

Average A-level requirements	• ABB at A-level plus a B at AS-level. Biology or chemistry must be AS-level if not taken at A-level
Average Scottish Higher requirements	• Require Advanced Highers, please check with school
Make-up of interview panel	• Three academic staff and senior student
Months in which interviews are held	• November–March
Proportion of overseas students	• 7.5%
Proportion of mature students	• 30%
Faculty's view of students taking a gap year	• Encouraged
Proportion of students taking intercalated degrees	• 30%
Possibility of direct entrance to clinical phase	• Oxbridge and students from other UK medical schools
Fees for graduates	• £1100
Fees for overseas students	• £11 535 pa (preclinical) and £20 225 pa (clinical)
Assistance for elective funding	• Yes (limited funding available)
Assistance for travel to attachments	• Limited reimbursement available
Access and hardship funds	• Yes
Weekly rent	• Halls £57.50 (non-catered), £80 (catered), Private £65
Pint of lager	• Union bar £1.30 City centre pub £2.00
Cinema	• £2–£7
Nightclub	• Free–£20 (easy access to London's West End)

Further information

St George's Hospital Medical School
Cranmer Terrace
London SW17 0RE
Tel: 0208 6729944
Email: adm-med@sghms.ac.uk
Web: http://www.sghms.ac.uk

Sheffield

Key facts	Sheffield
Course length	5 years
Total number of medical undergraduates	1000
Applicants in 2002	2400
Interviews given in 2002	42%
Places available in 2002	238
Places available in 2003	238
Entrance requirements	ABB
Mandatory subjects	Chemistry + another science subject
Male:female ratio	1:1.7
Premed course	Yes
Fast-track course	No

Sheffield is a city built – like Rome – on seven hills, and is almost, but not quite, as scenic! The university has a very large undergraduate population (15 000+) and Sheffield is reputedly one of the best student cities in Britain (see *The Virgin Alternative Guide to British Universities*), and that includes the big place down south. It was given the title of UK University of the Year for 2001. The majority of students live and work in the scenic or, in other words, hilly parts of town, but there is a wide variety of areas to choose from. The medical school attracts students from all walks of life and there is a good mixture of backgrounds. It uses a systems-based teaching scheme, running since 1994, which is under regular review. In general the curriculum can be looked upon as being a hybrid of the traditional science-based course and the newer problem-based approach, with increasing emphasis on self-directed learning. There tends to be one set of exams at the end of each year, and some project work is undertaken in groups throughout the year.

Education

The course is divided into six phases. Phases Ia and b are essentially the first and second years. Phase II lasts for only six months and involves an introduction to clinical medicine. The phase finishes with a set of objective structured clinical exams or OSCEs in January. There are no written papers at the end of this phase. Phases IIIa and b follow this and last two years. Phase IIIa is assessed with both OSCEs and written exams. At the end of Phase IIIb you sit your final written papers, for the MBChB. Phase IV starts with six months of purely clinical work, and the final OSCEs for the MBChB are taken in the summer.

The clinical course has been redesigned to increase the number of ward attachments, but the time spent on each attachment has had to shorten. These changes have given students a broader range of experience and teaching, but have reduced the opportunity to settle into a placement.

Teaching

The emphasis at Sheffield is on teaching broad concepts rather than detailed facts. This relies on the students' desire to look things up for themselves, and hopefully produces doctors who are committed to lifelong learning. There is a lot of anatomy dissection, with plenty of opportunity to get "hands-on" experience, as well as practicals in physiology and biochemistry. Animals are not used in the laboratory, although animal products are. The number of lectures has been reduced to allow time for small group project work and self-directed learning. Clinical years consist mostly of ward-based attachments, interspersed with lecture blocks and tutorials in the third year.

Assessment

Assessment of preclinical students is mainly by the end-of-year exams, which comprise written multiple-choice papers and practical spotter exams. The practical exam consists of dissection specimens to test anatomy, physiology, biochemistry, and physiology, but there is also some continuous assessment through projects and practical write-ups. There are also brief anonymous tests at the end of each module, which are used as a means to monitor your own progress – otherwise known as formative assessment. In the clinical years OSCEs are added as well as written papers, and are used to examine clinical skills.

Intercalated degrees

The option of spending an extra year studying for a Bachelor of Medical Science (BMedSci) is open to anyone who has passed all their preclinical exams. Funding is available for most places, which are generally research and/or laboratory based. There is little competition for places and students can "design" their own degree. The faculty publishes a list of projects open to BMedSci students, and staff tend to be very keen to recruit students.

Special study modules and electives

There is one eight-week elective period during the fourth year. Attachments (if approved by faculty) are usually completed abroad. Some help with funding is available. Also, many clinical students get involved in their own special study modules (SSMs) by helping a relevant consultant in their chosen expertise, either as research, audit, or the like.

Facilities

Library   Libraries are sited around the university and in all hospitals used for teaching. The two main medical libraries have been refurbished and have on-site computer access, including access to the internet and Medline. Core texts and places to sit are increasing, but be prepared to fight for them at exam time. Opening hours are reasonable, but are limited during weekends.

Computers   There are widespread computer facilities throughout the university and in the Royal Hallamshire, but be prepared to wait at peak times. One site is open 24 hours. Software provided includes email, internet access, and an increasing number of computer-assisted learning packages which students are encouraged to use.

Clinical skills   There are two new laboratories, one at the Northern General and one at the Royal Hallamshire.

Welfare

Student support

First-year students are eased into the course fairly gently, and there are usually plenty of people around to help you with problems. Most lecturers are willing to help solve academic problems, and the Undergraduate Dean is very approachable. Each student is allocated a social tutor, and medical students from the years above as part of a social group to help out with any problems and offer advice, but the scheme tends to be patchy, depending on the involvement of individual tutors. It is currently under review. The Students' Union and the university have counsellors and welfare support. A new "buddy scheme" has been initiated whereby a couple of medical students in the second year act as "parents" for a couple of students in the year below. The point of this is not, as it may at first seem, to be an extension of the nanny state! Instead, it serves to provide a source of information, help, and so on for first-years in case they are unwilling to approach academic staff.

Accommodation

All first-years are guaranteed university-owned accommodation, either in a catered hall of residence or in self-catering accommodation. The standard is pretty good, a major plus being that it is all within easy walking distance of university and in the better part of town. Most (but not all) students move into the private rented sector for their second year. Plenty of housing is available, mostly on 12-month contracts.

Placements

The medical school is based at the Royal Hallamshire Hospital, which is situated adjacent to the main university campus. Preclinical teaching takes place mainly at the medical school, the biomedical sciences building, the auditorium within the university Union, and in other parts of the main university site, mainly in the biomedical sciences department. The clinical years are taught on the wards of the various Sheffield and district general hospitals. Lecture blocks for the whole year group are held in the medical school and the excellent Union cinema (!), but smaller groups attend the Northern General Hospital Education Centre. This provides much better teaching facilities, but is situated on the other side of town (20 minutes from the university).

There are five hospitals in the centre of Sheffield, including the two extremely large teaching hospitals – the Northern General and the Royal Hallamshire – and the Sheffield Children's Hospital. The other two are the Weston Park Hospital, specifically for cancer patients, and the newly built Jessops Wing for women at the Royal Hallamshire.

Throughout the clinical phase there are peripheral attachments in hospitals throughout South Yorkshire and Humberside (up to 50 miles away). There is also an eight-week attachment at a GP practice in or around Sheffield, to which students commute. First-year students shadow a patient suffering from a chronic illness, to assess the impact of disease on daily living. This is known as the community attachment scheme (CAS), and takes a different approach to most of the medical course because of its emphasis on the social effects of disease, rather than how to treat it. Clinical skills, such as history taking from actual patients, are included from the first year onwards. A new, unique feature of the first year is that following the Christmas vacation there is a three-week block consisting of early patient contact with a doctor, nurse, and nursing home staff in separate one-week blocks. This is called intensive clinical experience (ICE).

Sports and social

City life

The city centre is compact and not terribly well formed, but has a good collection of small shops and restaurants, and Division Street has lots of trendy student shops and many trendy bars. Eccleshall Road boasts many trendy cafés and shops but is situated in the more scenic part of Sheffield, not far from the centre. (Real shopaholics go to the huge purpose-built out-of-town Meadowhall Centre, accessible by bus, train, and tram, which contains every high-street store under the sun.) Sheffield is famous for having the most bars and pubs in one city outside London. There is an ever-increasing number of new nightclubs, café-bars, and live music venues. As there are lots of clubs there is a student night nearly every day of the week, with cheap entry, drinks promotions, and a free bus to and from the venue. There are two theatres and five cinemas which all have student discounts for those after a bit of culture: the UGC cinema contains the biggest screen in Europe, appropriately called "The Full Monty". The crowning glory of Sheffield is the Peak District. This attracts many active outdoor types (especially climbers) to the university, as well as those who like to relax over a pint in a nice country pub. Just 10 minutes' drive from the university you can walk, cycle, climb, admire the stunning scenery, and forget about medicine. The locals are generally cheery and it is very easy to settle in at Sheffield quickly.

Uni life

The Medical Society organises regular social events: the annual November ball (be prepared to save up for it), and the legendary medics' revue are particularly well supported, as well as the annual fancy dress three-legged pub crawl and loads of lectures involving free pizza. If you would rather bypass medics after working hours, there are clubs for every taste and style, including Gatecrasher, Republic, Poo Na Na, Kingdom, National Centre for Popular Music, The Leadmill, and the ever more popular NY Sushi. The Students' Union organises cheap and cheerful events every night of the week, including Pop Tarts if you like your culture "dumbed down". There is a huge variety of clubs and societies available to join: anyone fancy the Warhammer Assassins' Guild, or Star Trek the Whistling Society? Those interested in the more altruistic side to medicine can join the Marrow Appeal set up by medical students, or the Medical Students' International Network (MedSIN), which are both active in Sheffield. In addition, people from all religious denominations are catered for through their respective religious societies. In particular, within the medical school and the Students' Union there are Muslim prayer rooms.

Sports life

The city of Sheffield has inherited a large range of world-class sports facilities after hosting the World Student Games, including the Olympic swimming pool at Pondsforge and Don Valley athletics stadium. Unfortunately, the free university facilities are on the disappointing side, consisting mainly of a pool and several Astroturf pitches. All sports are well catered for, but the dry ski slope and indoor climbing wall are particular attractions. The medical school has numerous sports teams, with the rugby, football, and hockey clubs all being particularly active.

Great things about Sheffield

- The course allows individuals to learn at their own pace. Lecturers are very accessible and are usually happy to help with any problems.
- There are still dissection and hands-on practicals instead of prosections, which are beginning to turn up in all new medical curricula. Definitely a dying breed.
- There are endless clubs for all music tastes, bars and coffee shops for the trendsetters, and just about every type of entertainment under the sun.
- Student accommodation is in the nicer parts of town, within easy (and safe) walking distance of the university and all local amenities. In 2001 Sheffield was voted the safest student city in the UK.
- Sheffield medics are down to earth and represent a wide cross-section of society. Medical students are part of the university as a whole, and not just the medical school. This enables them to make use of all the facilities available, and to escape from medicine when they want to.

Bad things about Sheffield

- Students complain of poor course organisation, and lack of up-to-date information on the continually changing curriculum.
- Self-directed learning is hard if you are a poor self-motivator and leave things to the last minute; with formal assessment only at the end of the year, it's easy to fall behind.

- According to the consultants, they don't teach anatomy like they used to ... or physiology, or biochemistry, etc ... .
- Some of the peripheral attachments are to slightly less than glamorous towns – Hull, Grimsby, Rotherham, Scunthorpe, Barnsley, etc.
- Hills – good practice if you're training for Everest!

Additional application information

Average A-level requirements	• ABB (AB in two science subjects, one of which must be chemistry)
Average Scottish Higher requirements	• AAAAB + Advanced Highers, A in chemistry and B in at least one other science
Make-up of interview panel	• Medically qualified member of staff, biomedical scientist, medical student
Months in which interviews are held	• Mid-November–mid-March
Proportion of overseas students	• 6%
Proportion of mature students	• N/A
Faculty's view of students taking a gap year	• Applicants not disadvantaged if gap year taken
Proportion of students taking intercalated degrees	• 7–8% per year
Possibility of direct entrance to clinical phase	• Yes, if places available
Fees for graduates	• £1100
Fees for overseas students	• £9300 (preclinical) £17 000 (clinical)
Assistance for elective funding	• Yes, bursaries and loans available
Assistance for travel to attachments	• No
Access and hardship funds	• Yes
Weekly rent	• Halls £49–£100 Private £40-£60
Pint of lager	• Union bar £1.30 City centre pub £2
Cinema	• £1.50–£3.80
Nightclub	• £3–£9

Further information

Sub-Dean for Admissions
Medical School
University of Sheffield
Beech Hill Road
Sheffield S10 2RX
Tel: 0114 271 1910
Fax: 0114 271 3961 or 3960
Email: rs@sheffield.ac.uk
Web: http://www.sheffield.ac.uk

Southampton

Key facts	Southampton
Course length	5 years
Total number of medical undergraduates	957
Applicants in 2002	2500
Interviews given in 2002	Only mature and overseas applicants are interviewed
Places available in 2002	200
Places available in 2003	200
Entrance requirements	AAB
Mandatory subjects	Chemistry
Male:female ratio	37:63
Premed course	No
Fast-track course	Commencing September 2004

The medical school at Southampton University is modern and student friendly. It is one of the youngest medical schools, with a well-developed modern course. Southampton pioneered the new integrated curriculum now in operation in most UK medical schools. As such, it has had more experience than most schools at settling in to the new ways of learning medicine. Plans exist to develop an innovative programme of interprofessional learning in conjunction with the School of Nursing and Midwifery and the School of Health Professions and Rehabilitation Sciences. Southampton has just about everything city life has to offer, but on a scale which is easy to cope with, and, of course, it's by the sea!

Education

The fully integrated course has an increasing clinical component throughout the five years. During the first two years, each term deals with the basic science and clinical aspects of a major organ system, and includes clinical sessions in general practice and in the labour ward. Year 3 is the first clinical year, and students work in the Southampton area. Exams at the end of this year integrate basic science and clinical knowledge, a feature that is valued by students. The fourth year comprises clinical experience in the minor specialties, plus a research project. This educational innovation enables students to study an area of their choice for eight months, finishing with a dissertation and presentation. Some are fascinated by their project, but others are not and feel they forget a lot of the first three years' teaching. Final-year students are spread throughout the Wessex region in large teaching hospitals and smaller district general hospitals. Southampton has complied with GMC recommendations to limit the amount of factual knowledge that is required, and as a result the examinations are not structured to make you regurgitate thousands of facts but to test your ability to solve clinical problems, that is, to be a good doctor!

Teaching

In the early years students spend most of their time on the main university campus with other, non-medical, students learning in lectures, tutorials, and laboratory practicals. Southampton has also been introducing computer-based learning into the curriculum.

Assessment

The major exams are at the end of years 1 and 3 and throughout the final year.

Intercalated degrees

Between 5% and 15% of students take the opportunity to spend an extra year between third and fourth years to study for a BSc in basic or social sciences. Only a few students do this, because of the extra expense and because all students spend time in research during the fourth year. Students who already have undergraduate research experience may skip the fourth-year project and take an accelerated course, qualifying six months earlier.

Special study modules and electives

At the end of the third year students have an eight-week elective during which they may decide to spend time working in a hospital abroad. There are special study modules during the third year, where students may choose to study a particular area in depth, and in the fifth year there is a five-week block when students choose which specialty to gain additional experience in.

Facilities

Library Students have access to the Biomedical Sciences Library on the main campus and the Health Sciences Library at the General Hospital. Library facilities are good, although the most popular books are always in demand and students find it more convenient to buy core texts.

Computers The computer facilities are very good and are updated regularly. Workstations are available all over the campus, at the General Hospital, and in some halls of residence.

Clinical skills   This is an excellent facility and used in the medicine in practice course in years 1 and 2, as well as in some of the clinical attachments in years 3 and 4, and for revision during final year.

Welfare

Student support

Most people are struck by the friendliness of the staff and students at the medical school when they visit. A scheme has recently been set up whereby students run minitutorials for newer students in order to pass on the most relevant information: which books to buy, books not to buy, consultants with nice yachts who often need crew on trips round the Channel Isles – all the really important stuff. Southampton University has a counselling service, and the Students' Union has welfare services.

Accommodation

Students will be offered a place in halls of residence for their first year only. There is a range of options, from a small self-catering room with no sink, to a large en-suite room with breakfast and evening meal. Which you choose is governed mostly by your bank balance! A limited number of places are available in halls for subsequent years, but most people move into private rented houses in the Highfield and Portswood areas. Most halls are within a mile of the medical school.

Placements

The main university campus is in the Highfield/Bassett area of Southampton and is close to most of the halls of residence. The General Hospital, where most of the third and fourth years as well as one or two days a week in years 1 and 2 are spent, is about one mile away in Shirley. There is a reliable university bus service connecting all sites.

Clinical attachments may be in local Southampton hospitals or, in the final year, in several hospitals in the region as far afield as Guildford or Portsmouth. In these final-year placements there are fewer students per hospital and, consequently, more individual attention; students give excellent feedback from these placements. Accommodation and travel expenses are provided on peripheral attachments.

Sports and social 🏆

City life

Southampton has been widely rebuilt, having been heavily bombed during the war. There is a wide range of shops and restaurants, and most of the amenities you would expect of a city are evident. There are over 35 000 students in the city, which has a range of clubs, pubs, cinemas, and eateries.

The New Forest is popular for nature lovers, cyclists and "pub-lunchers", and the Solent and the Isle of Wight are popular with sailors. The proximity to Bournemouth beach is a bonus for sun and sand lovers. London is close enough for a day or night out by car, coach, or train.

Uni life

The Students' Union runs every club you could ever imagine wanting to join, and quite a few others besides! The Union building hosts nightclub events and bands. The on-site theatre and concert hall host lots of non-mainstream acts and performances. The medical school is renowned for its strong social life, and has a number of sporting and other societies. There is an annual ball, which is the most popular in the university, and an extravagant Christmas revue, which never fails to entertain.

Sports life

The University of Southampton has excellent watersports teams. The facilities are accessible to everyone, from those who have never sailed/rowed/canoed in their lives to those who wish to compete at an international level. Southampton has teams in most sports.

Great things about Southampton

- Excellent course which is well liked by students.
- Good patient/doctor to student ratio on attachments.
- Students are part of the main university, not just the medical school.
- All staff are very student friendly and approachable and there is a great support network for any problems.
- It's on the south coast, therefore the warmest – and it's by the sea!

Bad things about Southampton

- As it's one of the newest medical schools, some of the older consultants tend to be sceptical about any "newfangled" ways of doing things.
- Too many distractions – university social life, medical school social life, good lectures, beautiful countryside.
- The city's nightlife isn't what it could be.
- Having the elective after just one year of clinical work makes you less useful in a hospital abroad.
- Some of the fifth-year attachments can leave you feeling isolated and away from Southampton (for example Isle of Wight), but this doesn't last too long – maximum eight weeks.

Additional application information

Average A-level requirements	• AAB, must include chemistry and one other science
Average Scottish Higher requirements	• Please check with the school
Make-up of interview panel	• Academic, clinician and lay person
Months in which interviews are held	• November–March
Proportion of overseas students	• 12% per intake
Proportion of mature students	• 25% per intake
Faculty's view of students taking a gap year	• Encouraged if used for work experience, voluntary service or travel
Proportion of students taking intercalated degrees	• 15%
Possibility of direct entrance to clinical phase	• No
Fees for graduates	• £1100
Fees for overseas students	• £10 460 pa (preclinical) and £19 285 pa (clinical)
Assistance for elective funding	• Limited bursaries available
Assistance for travel to attachments	• Some
Access and hardship funds	• Yes
Weekly rent	• Halls £48–£93 Private £50
Pint of lager	• Union bar £1.40 City centre pub £2
Cinema	• £2–£5
Nightclub	• Free–£8

Further information

Admissions Office
University of Southampton
Biomedical Sciences Building
Bassett Crescent Building
Bassett Crescent East
Southampton SO15 7FX
Tel: 02380 594408
Fax: 02380 594159
Email: prospenq@soton.ac.uk
Web: http://www.som.soton.ac.uk/

Wales (Cardiff)

Key facts	Cardiff
Course length	5 years
Total number of medical undergraduates	1243
Applicants in 2002	1500
Interviews given in 2002	60%
Places available in 2002	304
Places available in 2003	304
Entrance requirements	370 UCAS tariff points, including ABB A-level
Mandatory subjects	Chemistry and biology at A or AS-level
Male:female ratio	40:60
Premed course	Yes
Fast-track course	In 2004

The University of Wales College of Medicine in Cardiff is a member college of the University of Wales responsible for the provision of teaching of medicine, dentistry, nursing, radiography, physiotherapy, occupational therapy, and other professions allied to medicine. This provides a unique opportunity for interprofessional health education, plus a Students' Union solely for these students. Increasing links and a proposed merger with Cardiff University will increase yet further the facilities available to medical students. The university has strong links with all hospitals in Wales, offering clinical placements across the Principality. Students from all walks of life – mature, overseas, Welsh and non-Welsh – make a varied student body, providing a peer group for almost any person. The university is ideally located for the leisure/recreation/social facilities available in this small, yet friendly capital city.

Education

The course has been following the new curriculum since October 1995. The new course is guided by five themes and delivered through 11 subject panels, with practical experience gained through clinical modules. Year 1 is the foundation year, introducing basic clinical and scientific skills and knowledge, with years 2 and 3 developing them further. Years 4 and 5 place a greater emphasis on clinical experience in preparing for the role of house officer. Teaching is provided through core and special study module components.

Teaching

A combination of lectures, tutorials, small group sessions, and self-directed learning makes up the bulk of the learning. Anatomy is learnt by hands-on human dissection and taught using demonstrated dissection and prosections. Various computer-assisted learning programs are used, mainly as a revision medium and for tutorial support. Firm sizes vary depending on the hospital: five to six in the main teaching hospitals, and usually two in the district general hospitals (DGHs) (varying from one to four).

Assessment

Examinations take place at the end of first, third, fourth, and fifth years, with resits being available in the first and third years. Continuous assessment and the satisfactory completion of all coursework and special study modules are a feature of the examination process.

Intercalated degrees

Intercalated degrees are available to one-third of the year, and can be done after years 2, 3, and 4. There is a choice of subjects, including basic medical sciences (anatomy, physiology, biochemistry), or more clinically orientated modular degrees in medical sciences.

Special study modules and electives

Special study modules make up 24–30% of the timetable throughout the five years. An eight-week period of elective study, either in the UK or abroad, is undertaken in the final year as part of the normal block rotation.

Facilities

Library The library facilities in the main teaching hospital consist of three separate libraries, two 24-hour reading rooms and a 40-PC 24-hour computer room. The availability of texts and journals is excellent. Students also have access to the library and computing facilities of the University of Wales, Cardiff University, and many other libraries in most hospitals.

Computers There are adequate computer facilities on site, and in most outlying hospitals. Some tuition is given initially, and all submitted work is expected to be wordprocessed.

Clinical skills Cardiff has a new skills laboratory which is heavily used. It is a key focus for the new curriculum.

Welfare

Student support

UWCM is very student friendly and actively encourages and acts upon the views of its students. Monthly meetings between year reps and the Dean occur where students' grievances are voiced in an informal setting. Students are also represented on all the curriculum planning committees. Being part of the University of Wales allows students access to its general counselling and welfare services, as well as pastoral care within the faculty.

Accommodation

Accommodation is provided in the first year by Cardiff University. There is space for all first-years in halls. The standards are high, with over 50% of accommodation being less than five years old, and two-thirds is en-suite. There is ample good-quality private housing for rent, with prices ranging from £45 to £55 a week. Cardiff Council runs a house renting registration scheme, which aims to monitor and license rented accommodation in the city.

Placements

The medical school is based on two sites approximately 1.5 miles apart: the Cardiff School of Biosciences (a part of Cardiff University) and UWCM at the University Hospital of Wales. Community-based teaching in practices in and around Cardiff forms a substantial part of the course. Hospitals throughout Wales are used for teaching, ensuring an excellent student–patient ratio. It also provides an opportunity for students to see all of the different parts of Wales, and gain more of an idea where to apply for jobs a few years down the line. Bangor is the most distant of the DGHs used, being 260 miles away from Cardiff. Attachments in general practice include some time spent at a rural practice somewhere in Wales. Travel subsidies are available from the college, and accommodation is provided in all DGHs outside Cardiff.

Sports and social

City life

Cardiff is a very student-friendly city. UWCM, Cardiff University, UW Institute Cardiff, and the Welsh College of Music and Drama combine to make a student population of over 26 000. Most clubs/pubs/theatres, etc. host student nights/special rates for NUS card holders. The city also has plenty of parks and open spaces, so there is always somewhere to relax and sunbathe, especially in the summer. As the capital, Cardiff has all the attractions that you would expect of a large city while being small enough to make you feel at home. The local countryside is very beautiful, and all outdoor activities are available. The development of Cardiff Bay and the Welsh Assembly has given added excitement to the atmosphere in the city.

Uni life

Medical students are members of their own Students' Club, which provides sporting facilities/teams, its own fleet of minibuses, and its own bar, where drinks are often the cheapest in Cardiff! The Students' Club organises three staff/student dinners a year, six balls, and many other social events, ranging from top-name bands, comedians, long-distance pub crawls, and tours around the UK – all attended by a mix of medics, dentists, nurses, radiographers, and physiotherapy students. A wide range of clubs and societies are available, including climbing, orchestra, canoeing, and martial arts. There are also religious groups such as the Islamic Society and the Christian Medical Fellowship. Each year the students organise a charity revue called 'Anaphylaxis' and *Medrag* to raise money for local charities. In 1992 the Students' Union started its own charity, BACCUP. Each year a limited number of UWCM students have the opportunity to travel out to Belarus to work in an orphanage for children with special needs. Students also have access to the much greater facilities provided by Cardiff University and its Students' Union.

Student life can be very hectic, juggling work commitments with the variety of sports and clubs offered by UWCM Students' Club. The majority of teams, clubs, and societies are fully funded by the Club, including the provision of five minibuses for the use of its members. 'Medclub', UWCM's own bar/club, provides a friendly/social/cheap venue for the post-match celebrations and a very cheap source of alcohol for those not partaking in the sporting scene! It is also the venue for some of the craziest scenes you're likely to find during freshers' week. There is also the impressive Cardiff Students' Union, with its two bars, 1800 capacity nightclub, live music venue, and snooker/pool hall. As a capital city, Cardiff also offers excellent sport, leisure, and recreational facilities. The Millennium Stadium hosts the FA Cup and the Worthington Cup Finals, the Six Nations rugby, as well as a number of live music gigs. Cardiff also has a great range of shops, pubs, clubs, and a redeveloped seafront at Cardiff Bay. Living in Cardiff also allows easy access to beautiful and varied scenery, including the Brecon Beacons National Park .

Sports life

The Club has a large number of teams, some of which gain great success far beyond that expected of a small university. Our rugby team has won the Medschools cup six out of the last seven years! Most teams compete in the various BUSA inter-university competitions, inter-medical school competitions, and some local leagues. The Students' Club also has a multigym, pool, and snooker tables. Besides the facilities on offer by the dedicated Students' Union of UWCM, students have the benefit of using the sports and Union facilities of Cardiff University.

Great things about Cardiff

- Students are members of the Students' Unions at UWC (Cardiff Uni) and UWCM, allowing access to both Medclub and the bars and nightclub at Cardiff Uni. This also allows medical students to socialise with non-medics as well as medics.

Wales (Cardiff)

- A lot of interactions (socially and academically!) between students of all years, and with dental, nursing, physios, etc.
- All the advantages of living in an expanding and vibrant capital city without the usual costs.
- Using all Welsh hospitals keeps firm sizes low and student/patient ratios high.
- An excellent course with one of the best balances between problem-based learning, lectures, and clinical experience.

Bad things about Cardiff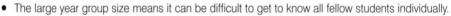

- The large year group size means it can be difficult to get to know all fellow students individually.
- The wait for coursework to be returned is often long.
- Distances between hospitals and the accessibility of some rural hospitals make travelling very awkward/time consuming, unless you have a car.
- Clinical placements in the fourth and fifth years can make it hard to see your non-medic friends (and medic friends not with you on placement) regularly.
- The weather!

Additional application information

Average A-level requirements	• Two science A-levels (chemistry, biology, physics, maths, statistics) at AB grades. Chemistry and biology to AS-level if not A-level (B grades). Non-science subjects encouraged, except general studies
Average Scottish Higher requirements	• AAAAB (including chemistry, biology, physics and English) & two Advanced Highers at AA incl. chemistry
Make-up of interview panel	• Mix of clinicians, GPs, scientists, lay people, staff in medically related fields (radiography, nursing, etc.) and medical students
Months in which interviews are held	• November–April
Proportion of overseas students	• 7.5%
Proportion of mature students	• 7%
Faculty's view of students taking a gap year	• No problem, provided there are plans to use the year constructively
Proportion of students taking intercalated degrees	• 20–33%
Possibility of direct entrance to clinical phase	• There must be strong personal reasons to transfer in and courses must be compatible
Fees for overseas students	• £9600 pa (preclinical) and £17 920 pa (clinical)
Assistance for elective funding	• Some small scholarships available
Assistance for travel to attachments	• Free transport provided in South Wales area, 50% of rail fare to mid/North Wales
Access and hardship funds	• Emergency loan funds and some grants available
Weekly	• Halls £44 standard £52 en-suite Private £45–£55
Pint of lager	• Union bar £1–£1.60 City centre pub £2.20
Cinema	• £3–£5.50
Nightclub	• Free–£5

Further information

Undergraduate Admissions Officer
University of Wales College of Medicine
Heath Park
Cardiff CF4 4XN
Tel: 029 2074 2027
Fax. 029 2074 2914
Email: uwcmadmissions@cf.ac.uk
Web: http://www.uwcm.ac.uk

Open days: February, April, June, July

Appendices

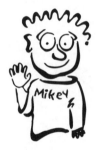

Mikey's quick compare table

Mikey's quick compare table

University	No. applicants (2002)	No. places (2002)	% interviewed	Entrance req.	Mandatory subject	M:F	% Intercalated year	% mature	% overseas	Fast track
Aberdeen	1214	175	66	ABB	Chemistry highly desirable	49:51	20	14	7	Yes
Belfast	551	181	7	AAB	Chemistry + another science	34:66	10	5	7	No
Birmingham	2097	340	33	AAB	Chemistry (Biology to AS)	45:55	15–20	3	10	
Brighton & Sussex				ABB	Biology/Chemistry	N/A	Provision to start in 2006			
Bristol	1757	230	40	AAB	Chemistry	41:59	30	15	5	Yes
Cambridge	1189	268		AAA	Chemistry and Biology	47:53	None	4	7	Yes
Dundee	1337	154	37	ABB	Chemistry	45:55	10	10	8	No
East Anglia	N/A	110	N/A	AAB	Biology	N/A	N/A		8	No
Edinburgh	2167	218	5	AAAB (3 A-levels, 1 AS)	Chemistry	35:65	40	3	8	No
Glasgow	1327	241	49	AAB	Chemistry	39:61	35	Varies	8	No
Guy's, King's and St Thomas'	3020	360	40	ABB	Chemistry and Biology (at least one to A-level)	39:61	50	Varies	8	Yes
Hull & York	N/A	130		ABB	Biology and Chemistry	N/A	Up to 15%	Up to 15%		No
Imperial	2500	326	41	ABB + A at AS-level	Biology and Chemistry	44:56	Built into the course	2.5	7	No
Leeds	1839	238	34	AAB	Chemistry	40:60	40–50	6	15 places/year	No
Leicester/Warwick	1400	175	60	AAB	Chemistry + Biology AS	45:55	5–10	10	7	Yes
Liverpool	1516	268	75	AAB	Chemistry and Biology (A or AS)	36:64	10	20	6	Yes

(Continued)

Mikey's quick compare table (continued)

University	No. applicants (2002)	No. places (2002)	% interviewed	Entrance req.	Mandatory subject	M:F	% Intercalated year	% mature	% overseas	Fast track
Manchester, Keele and Preston	1920	340	43	AAB	Chemistry	42:58	20–30 students each year	10		No
Newcastle and UDSC	1326	220	56	AAB	Chemistry or Biology	35:65	10	8	6	
Nottingham	<2000	245	20	AAB	Chemistry and Biology	35:65	All students do a BMedSci degree without an extra year	10	10	Yes
Oxford	788	150	93	AAA	Chemistry	45:55	100 – the Honours degree is mandatory			Yes
Peninsula	N/A	127	N/A	N/A	1 Science	N/A				No
Royal Free & UCL	<2300	330	50	ABB	Chemistry + Biology at A or AS level	45:55	Compulsory	12	7	No
St Andrew's	492	112		ABB	Chemistry	49:51	20	10	8.5	No
St Bart's & Royal London	1900	254	47	ABB	Chemistry or Biology	47:53	50	21	13	Yes
St George's	1551	190	4.7	ABB	Chemistry and Biology	52:48	30	30	7.5	Yes
Sheffield	2400	238	42	ABB	Chemistry + another science	35:65	7–8		6	No
Southampton	2500	200	Only mature/overseas applicants interviewed	AAB	Chemistry		15	25	12	
Wales (Cardiff)	1500	304	60	ABB	Chemistry and Biology	40:60	20–33	7	7.5	In 2004

Glossary

Medicine is full of jargon and abbreviations. Estimates suggest that students' vocabularies double over the course of a five-year medical degree. Unfortunately, it is such a part of life for medical students and doctors that they sometimes forget to speak in plain language to the general public. The following is a very brief list of words pertaining to medical education that you are likely to come across in this guide, and perhaps in medical school prospectuses. Our apologies for any jargon we have used in the guide not listed here!

Anatomy: The study of the structure of the body. Although this used to be taught by dissection, prosections (predissected specimens) are more commonly used nowadays.

Attachment: The term given to clinical placements. The student is placed under the supervision and guidance of a hospital consultant and his/her team (firm) or a GP for a period in the course.

Biochemistry: The study of the structure and functioning of the body at the molecular level.

British Medical Association (BMA): The doctors' professional association and trade union, providing representation and services for doctors and medical students.

BSc (Honours): see Intercalated degrees.

Clerking: Taking a history from and examining a patient on admission. A very useful learning experience if you are the first person to see the patient.

Computer-assisted learning (CAL): Computer programs are sometimes used to teach a topic in a more interactive format than a lecture/tutorial, and let the student set his/her own learning pace. They may also give the opportunity for self-assessment on a topic.

Consultant: The senior specialist doctor, usually based in a hospital.

Core curriculum: Under GMC directives the medical course is split into a core curriculum (in which all students must cover the same key topics to a high standard) and special study modules (in which the student can go in his/her own direction and study an area of interest in more depth) which may not be covered by all students.

District general hospital (DGH): A regional hospital which treats a broad spectrum of patients but refers more specialist cases to a teaching hospital. Medical students are taught by NHS staff, not university-employed consultants and registrars.

Elective: A period (usually 6–12 weeks in the latter years of the course) when students can choose an area of interest to study independently outside their medical school, either in the UK or, more often, abroad.

Endocrinology: The study of the hormonal function of the body.

Epidemiology: The study of the pattern and causes of diseases in society.

Firm: see Attachment.

General Medical Council (GMC): All medical degree courses must be approved by the GMC. It is the medical profession's self-regulatory body, which ensures professional standards are maintained and patients are protected. Doctors must be registered with the GMC to practise in the UK.

Honours year: see Intercalated degrees.

Integrated courses: Integration is the merging of several disciplines into one (hopefully more meaningful) course. Integration may be partial, within a single year or phase (for example, combining anatomy, physiology and biochemistry to teach body systems – respiratory, cardiovascular, reproduction, etc.), or it may be full, across all years, starting clinical teaching with basic medical sciences from the outset.

Intercalated degrees: Most schools offer students the opportunity to take an extra year (or two) in the middle of the course to study a subject of interest, leading to a BSc (Hons) or equivalent at the end. Some schools only offer this to high achievers, whereas others have an intercalated BSc (Hons) built into the course for everyone.

MBBS: The degree awarded to medical school graduates. (This varies slightly between schools, for example MBChB, MBBChir, but all are equivalent.)

Medical microbiology: The study of microorganisms and the diseases they cause.

Medline: A widely used and comprehensive computer database of articles published in medical journals.

Objective structured clinical examination (OSCE): A relatively new form of assessment where the students are set several tasks – taking histories, examining patients or performing tests/procedures – to complete in front of the examiner within a set time. The student is marked according to a standardised marking scheme. Every student is thus assessed identically, ensuring fairness and comparability of results between individuals.

Pathology: The study of disease processes and their effect on the structure and function of the body.

Peripheral attachments: Placements in hospitals/general practices outside the university area and normally outside the university town.

Pharmacology: The study of the action of drugs and their application.

Physiology: The study of the functioning of body systems and tissues.

Premedical year: Students without the necessary science entrance qualifications can apply to do a premedical year which takes them to a sufficient level of scientific knowledge to join the medical course the following academic year (not offered at all schools).

Preregistration house officer (PRHO): A newly qualified doctor working in the first year after graduation. House officers, despite being able to call themselves doctors and prescribe drugs, are provisionally registered by the GMC until they have completed this year satisfactorily. After this they achieve full registration.

Problem-based learning (PBL): Students learn from researching and solving a relevant (usually clinical) scenario, rather than being given all the information passively. Small group problem-solving tutorials, facilitated by members of staff, take the place of lectures.

Prosections: Predissected cadaver specimens of the human body used to teach anatomy. In many schools these have replaced actual dissection by students themselves.

Registrar: A doctor who is undergoing specialist training (usually for between three and nine years) before becoming a consultant or general practitioner. The next step up the ladder after SHO.

Self-directed learning: Learning under the student's own initiative from lists of objectives rather than didactic teaching (such as lectures).

Senior house officer (SHO): A junior hospital doctor who has completed his/her year as house officer.

Special study modules (SSMs): Periods of the course when students study areas of interest outside the core curriculum (see above). These may be taught or may be independent research projects.

Teaching hospitals: Normally the main hospital(s) in the university town or city. Services provided are part of the NHS, but the senior clinical staff will often be employed by the university and hold medical academic posts. Teaching hospitals usually handle specialist cases, which can be referred to them from DGHs across the region. Many such hospitals will have regional centres for particular specialties or centres of excellence, such as cardiology, plastic surgery, neonatal intensive care, etc.

Viva: An oral examination (sometimes referred to as a viva voce).

Abbreviations

BMA:	British Medical Association
CAL:	Computer-assisted learning
CSYS:	Certificate of sixth-year study (Scottish students)
DGH:	District general hospital
GMC:	General Medical Council
OSCE:	Objective structured clinical examination
PBL:	Problem-based learning
PRHO:	Preregistration house officer
SHO:	Senior house officer
SSM:	Special study module
UCAS:	Universities and Colleges Admissions Service

Further information

British Medical Association

The British Medical Association (BMA) is both the doctors' professional organisation and their trade union, protecting the professional and personal interests of its members. It is the voice of the medical profession in the UK and represents the profession internationally. Members and staff are in constant touch with ministers, government departments, Members of Parliament, and other influential bodies, conveying to them the profession's views on healthcare and health policy. Most medical students and practising doctors are members.

The BMA's head office is in London, and there are national offices in Scotland, Northern Ireland, and Wales. There are an additional 15 regional offices throughout the UK. The BMA is a medical publisher in its own right, but also includes the BMJ Publishing Group. The BMJ Publishing Group is a major medical and scientific publisher and publishes the weekly *British Medical Journal* and the monthly *Student BMJ*.

The Medical Students Committee (MSC) represents students within the Association and also to important outside bodies, such as the Departments of Education and Health and the General Medical Council. Through the committee the BMA campaigns on many issues, such as student finances and debt, reforms of the medical degree syllabus, and health and safety. Following devolution the BMA has established MSCs in Northern Ireland, Scotland, and Wales. There are student representatives and BMA committees in every medical school, and the BMA runs many local events and talks for students. The vast majority of medical students join the BMA.

Medical students who are members of the BMA receive a variety of benefits, including a free subscription to *Student BMJ*, free guidance notes, a free copy of *Clinical Evidence*, library and information services, and book discounts to name but a few. General information, guidance, and student chat board can be found on the BMA's Medical Students Committee website.

Medical Students Committee
British Medical Association   Tel: 020 7387 4499
BMA House   Fax: 020 7383 6494
Tavistock Square   Email: students@bma.org.uk
London WC1H 9JP   Web: http://www.bma.org.uk/students

Becoming a doctor

General information on getting into medical schools is available from the BMA website. *Medical Careers: a General Guide* (3rd revised edition): this publication is available free of charge to BMA members from their local BMA office, or at £10 to non-members from the BMJ Bookshop. Tel: 020 7383 6244.

Student BMJ

The *Student BMJ* is an international journal specifically for medical students. It is published monthly and includes articles on education, medical careers, student life, science, and news. Many of the articles and papers are written by medical students. Individuals or schools and libraries can subscribe to the journal.

For more information or a sample copy contact:

Student BMJ
BMJ Publishing Group
BMA House
Tavistock Square
London WC1H WR

Tel: 020 7383 6402
Fax: 020 7383 6270
Email: bmjsubs@dial.pipex.com
Web: http://www.studentbmj.com

Universities and Colleges Admissions Service (UCAS)

Universities and Colleges
Admissions Service
Rose Hill
New Barn Lane
Cheltenham
Gloucestershire GL52 3LZ

Tel: 01242 222444
Web: http://www.ucas.com

* *UCAS Handbook and Application Pack:* essential reading and material for applicants to university courses.

National Union of Students (NUS)

For general information on financial matters for students.

National Union of Students
Nelson Mandela House
Holloway Road
London N7 6LJ

Tel: 020 7272 8900
Fax: 020 7263 5713
Email: nusuk@nus.org.uk
Web: http://www.nusonline.co.uk

Department for Education and Skills

Web: http://www.dfes.gov.uk/studentsupport

The Scottish Office

There are many publications about higher education and funding for Scottish students available on the web or from:

The Stationery Office   Tel: 0131 228 4181 71
Lothian Road   Fax: 0131 622 7017
Edinburgh EH3 9AZ   Web: http://www.scotland.gov.uk

Charities

Copies of the following books should be available in the reference section of most public libraries:

- *The Charities Digest* – published by the Family Welfare Association
- *Money to Study* – published by UKOSA/NUS/EGAS
- *The Educational Grants Directory* – published by the Directory of Social Change
- *Directory of Grant-Making Trusts* – published by Charities Aid Foundation/Biblios.

The British Medical Association Charities Office (see BMA address) has information about awards and grants for mature and second degree medical students.

Christian Medical Fellowship (CMF)

Dr Mark Pickering   Tel: 020 7928 4694
Student Secretary   Fax: 020 7620 2453
Christian Medical Fellowship Email: student@cmf.org.uk or admin@cmf.org.uk
157 Waterloo Road   Web: http://www.cmf.org.uk
London SE1 8XN

CMF has over 5500 medical student and doctor members throughout the UK and Ireland. It exists to encourage fellowship, Christian ethics, evangelism, and medical mission, and to provide a Christian voice on medical issues. CMF runs conferences, coordinates local groups, and publishes widely at the interface of Christianity and medicine. It is one of 60 member bodies of the International Christian Medical and Dental Association (ICMDA). A publications catalogue and information about local groups, conferences, and activities are available from the above address.

Medical Students International Network (MedSIN)

Founded in 1997, MedSIN is an independent, student-run organisation which aims to facilitate medical students' involvement in humanitarian and educational activities at local, national, and international level. MedSIN groups in medical schools carry out sex education projects, international exchanges, bone marrow registration drives, seminars on topical issues, and much more. Through its membership of the International Federation of Medical Students' Associations (IFMSA), MedSIN also provides opportunities to go on projects all over the world, from Angola to Zimbabwe. The IFMSA was founded in 1951 and promotes international cooperation on professional training and the achievement of humanitarian ideals. To get in touch or find out more, visit the MedSIN website: http://www.medsin.org

Gay and Lesbian Association of Doctors and Dentists (GLADD)

GLADD was formed in 1995. It has an active student section and provides professional support, educational and social meetings, both locally and nationally. GLADD campaigns vigorously within the health service and in the country at large on issues of equality relating to the lesbian, gay, and bisexual community.

Email: gladd@dircon.co.uk
Web: http://www.gladd.dircon.co.uk

Armed forces: cadet recruitment

Army
Royal Army Medical Corps   Tel: 01276 412730
Recruiting Office   Fax: 01276 412731
Regimental Headquarters   Email: ramc.recruiting@army.mod.uk.net
Army Medical Services
Slim Road
Camberley
Surrey GU14 4NP

RAF
Medical and Dental Liaison Officer   Tel: 01400 261201 ext 6811
Directorate of Recruiting and   Fax: 01400 262220
Selection (Royal Air Force)   Email: mdlo@royalairforce.net
PO Box 100
Cranwell
Sleaford
Lincolnshire NG34 8GZ

Royal Navy
Med Pers (N)2   Tel: 02392 727818
Room 133   Fax: 02392 727805
Victory Building
HM Naval Base
Portsmouth PO1 3LS

Financial information

Financial arrangements and support vary depending on which country you intend studying in. Some support is provided by Departments of Education and Skills, and some from Departments of Health.

The Educational Grants Advisory Service provides information about student support systems in the UK and can help identify additional sources of funding.

Family Welfare Association   Tel: 0207 254 6251 (opening hours: Mondays,
501–505 Kingsland Road   Wednesdays, and Fridays 10 am–12 pm, and 2 pm–4 pm)
London E8 4AU   Email: egas.enquiry@fwa.org.uk
     Web: http://www.egas-online.org.uk

Relevant contact information for each nation is below.

England

For information and guides on student support ring the Department for Education and Skills (DFES).
Helpline: 0800 731 9133
Web: http://www.dfes.gov.uk

Financial Help for Health Care Students, a booklet by the Department of Health, explains NHS funding in more detail. Order one or download from the website:

Department of Health   Tel: 0845 60 60 655
PO Box 777   Email: doh@prologistics.co.uk
London SE1 6XH   Web: http://www.doh.gov.uk/hcsmain.htm

You can obtain bursary information from:

NHS Student Grants Unit   Tel: 01253 655655
22 Plymouth Road   Fax: 01253 206 1499
Blackpool FY3 7JS   Email: nhs-sgu@ukonline.co.uk

Scotland

Student Awards Agency for Scotland   Tel: 0131 476 8227
3 Redheughs Rigg   Web: http://www.student-support-saas.gov.uk/
South Gyle
Edinburgh EH12 9YT

Wales

Further and Higher Education Division of the National Assembly for Wales
Tel: 02920 825 831
Web: http://www.learning.wales.gov.uk

You can obtain bursary information from:

NHS Wales Student Awards Unit   Tel: 02920 261 495
2nd Floor Golate House
101 St Mary's St
Cardiff CF10 1DX

Northern Ireland

Information for students from Northern Ireland can be obtained from the Department for Employment and Learning:

Web: http://www.delni.gov.uk

Also try:

The Department of Health,   Tel: 02890 524746
Social Services and Public Safety   Web: http://www.dhsspsni.gov.uk
Human Resources Directorate

Further reading

- *Learning Medicine* by Peter Richards (formerly Dean of St Mary's Medical School) and Simon Stockill, published by BMJ Publishing Group and updated regularly. Now in its 16th edition, this title is available from the BMJ Bookshop. Price £13.95 (discount available for BMA members). Tel: 020 7383 6244. Web: http://www.bmjbookshop.com